THE DARK NIGHT OF THE SHED

Men, the mid-life crisis,
spirituality & sheds

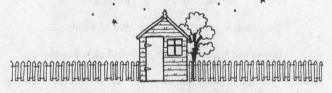

NICK PAGE

HODDER

Scripture quotations are from the New Revised Standard Version
of the Bible, © copyright 1989, 1995 by the Division of Christian
Education of the National Council of Churches of Christ in the United
States of America and are by permission. All rights reserved.

First published in Great Britain in 2015 by Hodder & Stoughton
An Hachette UK company

First published in paperback in 2016

1

A CIP catalogue record for this title is available from the British Library

ISBN 978 1 473 61685 1
eBook ISBN 978 1 473 61684 4

155.6081I

Typeset in Sabon by Hewer Text UK Ltd, Edinburgh

Printed and bound in the UK by Clays Ltd, St Ives plc

Hodder & Stoughton policy is to use papers that are natural, renewable
and recyclable products and made from wood grown in sustainable
forests. The logging and manufacturing processes are expected to
conform to the environmental regulations of the country of origin.

Hodder & Stoughton Ltd
Carmelite House
50 Victoria Embankment
London EC4Y 0DZ

www.hodderfaith.com

'I have to say I loved it, I love Nick Page's writing, I love his humour . . . he's got some very serious points to make which are particularly relevant to men, but to anyone really'
Clare Balding, BBC Radio 2

'a vulnerable, honest and amusing exploration of why many men have so much and yet feel like failures'
Harry Farley, *Christian Today*

'knowledge from psychology, especially Jung, sociology, and popular culture, is expressed in an always readable, informative way'
Church Times

'If I had to choose an author to sit in a pub with, put the world to rights, enjoy a beer, share a few jokes and prod the hairy subject of God and the male midlife crisis with a stick, there are few I'd choose over Nick Page . . . Few other books can provide that sense of a journey, genuinely do-able devotional suggestions, Biblical insight, lessons from Old Testament heroes and Percy the Park Keeper, generously inter-spersed with wit, good humour and some healthy self-deprecation'
Russ Bravo, *Inspire Magazine*

'An amusing book, but one with a profound message worth attending to'
The Irish Catholic

'A funny but insightful book about mid-life crisis in men . . . this new book deserves a wider readership'
The Church Newspaper

'A witty, deep book . . . One to buy as an early Christmas present for a man in your life'
Woman Alive Magazine

'If you are a man in your 40s or 50s, this is a book for you . . . Page brings humour to the situation and offers us solace'
The Methodist Recorder

'Nick Page is a very funny writer . . . I'd gladly recommend this to others. It's a very easy and enjoyable read . . . Honest and amusing'
Families First

CONTENTS

CONTENTS

INTRODUCTION

THE DARK NIGHT OF THE SHED

The vision

The night was dark. Cold.

I had woken suddenly, as so often, with a swarm of thoughts buzzing around my head. The usual greatest hits package of my fears and failures on repeat. I knew that it would be pointless trying to get back to sleep.

Instead, I got out of bed and walked across to the window. Looked out. The moon was full. The autumn leaves were rustling in the wind. There was a chill in the air.

Life as a middle-aged man had become complicated and confusing. At the time when I felt as though I should be confident and assured, I often felt anxious and afraid. I seemed to be dog-tired and exhausted, yet my nights were restless and disturbed. Aches and pains which used to disappear quite quickly now hung around for months. I carried within me a simmering pot of grumpiness which boiled over at the slightest excuse.

At the same time, I knew that something was happening within me, something was changing. I knew that I was entering a time of growth, setting out on a new adventure. It was a curious thing, but I felt both more fragile and yet stronger than ever before. That day I had started to plan a book about this journey. I wanted to talk about the things

I had learnt, all the men I had met. I wanted to explore the dark night I had been through, and, to a certain extent, was still in. But it wasn't working. Something was wrong. I couldn't quite find the right words.

It was then that I had my vision. I knew what would solve things. I knew with piercing, laser-focused certainty what I needed to make all things right.

I needed a shed. A really, really good shed.

Behind me, there was a sigh.

'It's two o'clock in the morning,' said The Wife sleepily. 'What are you doing?'

'I'm thinking about the shed,' I replied.

There was a pause.

'Of course you are,' she said.

I nodded. She understood. It all made perfect sense.

The next morning the whole shed idea looked slightly less visionary.

I had explained my brilliant insight several times now, to bemused looks from The Wife, the children and even the dog, and they had pointed out one major flaw in the whole 'I'm going to build a shed' idea, namely the fact that I already had one.

'Ah,' I replied, 'but do I *really* have one? Really?'

There was a pause.

'Yes,' said The Wife. 'It's just there.' She pointed out of the kitchen window to the shed which stood, literally, three yards from the back door.

'Yes, yes, I know there is *a* shed in the garden,' I replied, 'but it's not *mine*, is it? It's full of other people's stuff. I can't even get into it. It's not a proper shed, just a kind of garden cupboard.'

The Wife sighed. 'This is that programme, isn't it . . .'

Sussed.

The night before I had watched one of the greatest TV programmes ever made: *Shed of the Year*. Yes, my friends, there really is such a programme, and it ranks with the great monuments of TV culture, right up there with Kenneth Clarke's *Civilisation*, David Attenborough's *Life on Earth* and *Percy the Park Keeper*. But as I watched the programme, with its parade of wonderful sheds, shacks and miscellaneous outbuildings, my delight was tinged with jealousy. Why didn't I have one of these magnificent buildings myself?

'OK, then,' I said. 'I won't built a new shed. I will bring that one back to full . . . er . . . sheddiness. I will give it a new sense of purpose.'

She looked at me.

'It's a *shed*,' she said. 'What purpose do you want it to have?'

I ignored her. Visionaries are always misunderstood. It was too late, anyway. I knew now what I must do. I would transform the grotty, run-down structure that was quietly rotting away just outside. I would strip it down and start again. I would breathe new life into those old planks. I would turn it into a place where I could write about my experiences and the experiences of others, and how – like the shed itself – we could find a new kind of life and purpose.

It would be a place of refuge, a place to write and think and reflect. If I could get the shed sorted, then everything would be OK.

Is that it?

I'll be honest. I've never really been into the whole 'male-ness' thing. I don't mean *masculinity*. Earring aside, I like to think that I am fairly masculine. I have a beard and ear hair. I like sports and beer and can never resist childish innuendo. But all that macho, tree-hugging, triathlon-run-ning stuff about 'what it means to be a man' generally leaves me cold. I was once given a book called *Manhood* and, once I'd stopped giggling, I put it down somewhere with the fixed intention of never finding it again. I have rejected many, many invitations to spend time in fields, or climb mountains, or hug trees and generally rediscover my maleness. My maleness doesn't need rediscovering, thank you very much. It might need a bit of reupholster-ing, but that's a different issue.

But I felt I had to write this book. Because something happens to men in mid-life. Something strange.

Exactly what happens, and when, varies from person to person. Taken generally, there seems to be no precise defi-nition of when middle age begins. Some doctors identify the menopause as a starting point, while sociologists talk about that moment when your children leave home or the death of one's parents. Psychiatrists talk about sudden feelings of anxiety, anger or failure, economists point to unemployability or career peaks, biologists mention ageing, greying hair. All seem to agree that an awareness of our own mortality has something to do with it.

And it affects people differently. Many men simply breeze through this period, sailing serenely into old age with a sense of confidence and satisfaction. That's fine. No, really, I'm very pleased for them. Delighted. Couldn't be more thrilled. The smug ba—

Anyway.

For many of us, though, middle age is a much more turbulent sea to navigate. We become acutely aware of the dark depths beneath us. Doubts and anxieties strike like sudden squalls – deep questions about who we are and what we want to be. We look ahead into the darkness and start to be fearful of how this voyage is going to turn out. We feel old, disregarded, scared and useless, as though somehow we've failed or we're no longer appreciated. There is a horrible sense that the ship is slowly sinking. It looks OK on the outside, but inside we're springing leaks all over the place.

And from somewhere far off, carried on the wind, comes the single defining question of middle age: 'Is that it?'

While experts may argue over the exact extent of the so-called mid-life crisis, studies show that in middle age – most typically in the forties and fifties – levels of happiness and life satisfaction dip to their lowest, and depression and psychological distress are at their height. Forty-five is the most common age for depression to be diagnosed. A recent report by the Office of National Statistics shows that male suicide rates are now at their highest since 2001. Men are three times more likely to commit suicide than women. The number of incidents has risen steadily since the recession of 2007, and the most at-risk age group is between 45 and 59.[1]

Anecdotally speaking, I meet many men who have experienced some sense of disruption in mid-life. For some this has resulted in full-blown depression, for others a more general sense of dissatisfaction or anxiety. Relationships fracture or even fall apart. Most feel that sense of wondering what has happened and what is yet to come. Even for those men who do not experience overt negative effects, there is still often a desire for change. To do something different.

Some of their stories are in this book. Incidentally, for ease of use, I have decided to call all these people Steve. I thought this would help, as most men of my age can't remember the names of our own families, let alone characters in a book. And I think it's right to preserve anonymity. I'm fine with cannibalising my own life for case studies, but my friends' lives are a different matter. Nevertheless, they are all real people. Or, at least, they seemed real at the time.

Anyway, the point is, I frequently meet men who are grappling with this stuff. One of them, in particular, I see every day, staring back at me from the mirror.

At some point everyone, male or female, has to address the issue of what their life is really all about. For men, I think that this mid-life stage is one of the points when we encounter this question most clearly. And how we answer this question is of profound importance not only to ourselves, but also to all those around us.

That's why I wanted to write this book.

It's for men of a certain age. And the women who have to live with them.

It's for anyone who has ever looked around them and said to themselves, 'Is that it?'

It's for anyone who knows what it is to wake at night and feel that sense of stomach-churning anxiety that life is somehow leaving them behind.

It's for the disappointed, the anxious, the grumpy.

It's for anyone who feels that what they really need in life is a truly great shed.

Most of all, this is a book for people who want to change. Because that, I believe, is what these feelings are really all about. All these issues and questions and desires are signposts, invitations to a different, happier, more fulfilled life.

Especially the one about the shed.

PART ONE

THE INVITATION

*Midway upon the journey of our life
I found myself within a forest dark,
For the straightforward pathway had been lost.*

Dante, *Inferno*

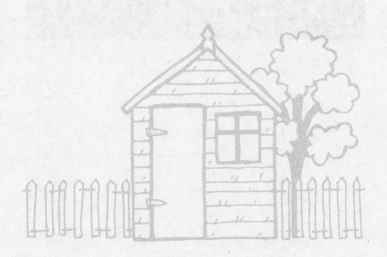

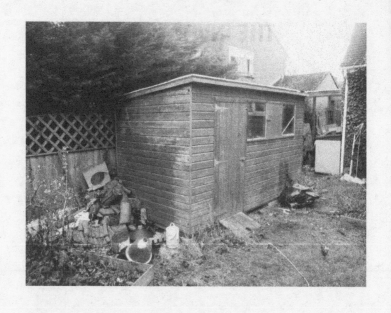

1

OF MEN, MIDDLE AGE AND SHEDS

The brotherhood of the shed

The family might have scoffed, but as the days went by and I started to plan and research, I realised just how stunningly insightful my vision had been.

First, there was the reaction of my male friends. When I told them of my plans to build the shed of my dreams, they didn't scoff. They nodded thoughtfully. Some grew tearful and could only give me a manly shake of the hand. They *understood*. I discovered Oxford Wood Recycling – an Aladdin's cave of pre-used timber, where I stocked up on hardboard for the floor. At one point I was joined at the pile of old boards by another man, tape measure in hand, and we divided the best bits between us.

'You building something?' he asked.

'A shed. Well, rebuilding it.'

'Me too.'

We nodded at each other. There was nothing more to say. We were shed brothers. In former lives we might have joined forces, roaming the ancient ridgeway and hunting a mammoth or two. Today we were hunting for the perfect bit of wood.

A brief history of sheds

Sheds have a long and magnificent history, it turns out. The Wife, showing either a surprisingly supportive nature or, more probably, taking the mickey, bought me a magnificent book called *The Joy of Sheds*. Author Frank Hopkinson has gathered together everything you could want to know about sheds, not to mention quite a lot that isn't worth knowing.

According to English Heritage, there are fifty-two Grade 2 listed sheds in England and Wales.[2] Even the name is appropriate. The word 'shed' comes from the Anglo-Saxon word *sceadu*, meaning 'shade', or 'comparative darkness' as the *Oxford English Dictionary* puts it. It comes from the same root as the word for 'shadow' (a word which we will be seeing more of later). It's the type of shade you find in a forest.* And what better place to think about the shadows of middle age than in the *sceadu* of a shed?

Sheds have had a massive impact on male culture. The Black & Decker Workmate® was invented in a shed. As were Ferodo tyres, Harley-Davidson motorcycles and Mercedes-Benz. Not to mention the Pot Noodle, which was cooked up, literally, in a shed by a Taiwanese inventor called Momofuku Ando. He was 61 at the time and lived to 96 – mainly on a diet of chicken noodles.

---

* 'Let us be Diana's foresters,' wrote Shakespeare, 'gentlemen of the shade.' That's in *Henry IV Part 1*, Act I, scene 2.26, in case you're interested.

For the writer, particularly, sheds are furnaces of creativity. There are the famous ones: Roald Dahl's writing
hut and George Bernard Shaw's revolving summerhouse,
the small octagonal hut just twelve feet across that Mark
Twain worked in. Philip Pullman wrote *Northern Lights*
in a shed. Daphne du Maurier wrote *My Cousin Rachel* in
a shed in the garden of her beloved Menabilly House in
Cornwall. Best of all, for a man of my generation, Oliver
Postgate and Peter Firmin created *Noggin the Nog*,
Bagpuss, *The Clangers* and *Ivor the Engine* in a shed
owned by Firmin. That one, surely, ought to be put on the
English Heritage list. Virginia Woolf used a converted
toolshed in her garden at Rodmell, Sussex. She called it a
Writing Lodge. It looked over the Ouse Valley. Sadly, it
was there that she wrote her last words in spring 1941,
before walking into the river, her coat pockets loaded
with stones. So, perhaps not the most encouraging
example.

I couldn't help noticing links between sheds and the
kind of stuff I wanted to explore in the book. When
Churchill was affected by what he called 'the black dog'
of depression, he would retreat to his shed to paint. The
troubled songwriter Nick Drake wrote a song called 'Man
in a Shed'. It's one of his cheerier numbers – which is not
saying a great deal – and as far as I can make out, it seems
to be about the danger of an inadequate shed roof. More
positively, Dylan Thomas wrote in a small 'wordsplashed
hut' overlooking the Taff Estuary. It was there that he
composed that theme tune to recalcitrant old age: 'Do not
go gentle into that good night.'

The King of Shed Writers, though, is Arthur Miller,
who, after the success of *All My Sons* on Broadway,

moved to a new house – and decided to build a shed to go with it. 'It was a purely instinctive act,' he later said. 'I had never built a building in my life.' As he built, he began to think about an idea for a play about a man whose dreams had never turned out to match the reality, and whose life was being torn apart. When he finally sat down at his desk (which he made from an old door), the play poured out of him. It was *Death of a Salesman* – of which more later.

Thoreau, one of my heroes, lived and wrote in a 10 foot by 15 foot hut of his own construction on the bank of Walden Pond in Connecticut. It was there, in 1845, that he wrote *Walden*, his classic of simple living. 'I went to the woods,' he wrote, 'because I wished to live deliberately, to front only the essential facts of life, and see if I could not learn what it had to teach, and not, when I came to die, discover that I had not lived.'[3] Surely this is the desire which drives the questions of mid-life. We want to know what life is for. We want to be sure that we have truly lived.

A brief history of middle age

Throughout the majority of human history the most pressing issue about middle age for most people was simply the challenge of living that long. Even as recently as 1900, the average life expectancy in Britain was about 47 for a man and 50 for a woman, although this figure is skewed because of the high rates of infant mortality. It was only later in the twentieth century that things changed. By the 1950s life expectancy had risen to about 65; by 1971 life expectancy for a man in Britain was 68 and for a woman, 72.[4] Today life expectancy at birth is 77 for a man in the UK and 81 for a woman and, according to some bloke on the radio I was just listening to, one in three of our children will live to be 100.

Middle age, though, is not a precise chronological event. It's more a state of mind. In fact the earliest mention of middle age comes from – well, the Middle Ages, actually. And it occurs in a poem which is all about the search for a meaningful life.

According to the *Oxford English Dictionary*, the first use of the term comes in 1400 in a poem called *Piers Plowman* by William Langland. The poem is all about the quest to find the true Christian life. It starts with the narrator falling asleep on the Malvern Hills (understandable: this is cider country). In the second half of the book, the narrator goes on a dream-quest to find the three figures who can tell him how to live. They are called Do-well, Do-better and Do-best. At one point the poet/dreamer is met by a figure representing imagination who, rather unimaginatively, is called 'Imagination'. He advises the narrator to 'make amends in middle age before your strength fails; for old age can ill endure the hardships of poverty and the life of penance and prayer'.[5]

This is the first use of the phrase 'middle age'. And, appropriately, it occurs in a story full of middle-aged stuff, a story which begins with the idea that life could be better, and is driven by the desire to find the real meaning of life. And most of all, it's a story that begins with a long nap.

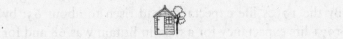

The Jung Ones

For the first serious analysis of the problems of middle age, we have to wait until the early twentieth century and the works of the psychologist Carl Jung.

Jung's work emerged from a mid-life crisis of his own. In July 1913, Jung turned 38. He was married, he had a family, he had professional status. His work in the relatively new field of psychotherapy had brought him to the attention of Sigmund Freud, who anointed Jung his spiritual heir. But all was not right in Jung's world. He had personal problems at home. And he had come to realise that he differed from Freud in some very significant ways. He could not pretend otherwise, even to his mentor. Freud could not countenance his disciple going in a different direction and there was an acrimonious split between the two. It plunged Jung into a kind of breakdown, which lasted four or five years. Jung described it as a 'confrontation with his unconscious' and later compared this period to the *nekyia* – Odysseus's visit to the land of the dead in Homer's *Odyssey*.

He became socially isolated and introspective. He had powerful dreams – sometimes disturbing, sometimes empowering. Yet it was a period which liberated him and led to his most influential ideas. 'It was then that I ceased to belong to myself alone, ceased to have a right to do so,' he wrote later. 'From then on my life belonged to the generality . . . I loved it and hated it, but it was my greatest wealth.'[6] He emerged more whole, more complete. In 1921 he published *Psychological Types*. And the following year he built a shed.

Well, I *say* a shed. A tower. A retreat. A small castle, in fact. In 1922 he bought some land by Lake Zürich at Bollingen, and on an outcrop built a simple round tower. He added to it over the course of his life. He had seen this tower in a dream when he was young and never forgot it. It was his place of refuge. And right in the middle of what became a suite of rooms, he had a room which was his alone, which only he was allowed to enter. 'At Bollingen I am in the midst of my true life, I am most deeply myself,' he wrote.[7]

In his influential essay *The Stages of Life*, Jung claimed that mid-life was a portal, a crucial stage in self-development. Jung believed there was a first and second half of life. Our 'youth' is the first half. According to Jung, this lasts until 'between the thirty-fifth and fortieth year'. In this part we are concerned with achievement, with building a career, a home, a useful place in society, with attaining our 'social goal'. We gather around us all the things which society says are important. In order to do this, we develop what Jung termed a *persona* – the face which we present to society. But our persona is not who we truly are. And sooner or later we have to come to terms with that.

That is the work of the second half of life. The second half of life is where we can – if we want – become a true, whole individual. Jung called this process 'individuation'. And the bit between the two halves of life – that is middle age.

In 1965, a psychologist called Elliot Jacques coined the term 'the mid-life crisis'. In a paper called 'Death and the Mid-life Crisis', Jacques examined the lives of over three hundred major artists, analysing their output before and after the ages of about 35 to 39. He observed that the 'hot from the fire' creativity of their youth was replaced by a more measured, 'sculpted creativity'. He concluded that the transformation was caused by a mid-life crisis, which was basically the sudden realisation that, sooner or later, you were going to pop your clogs.

Jacques' phrase caught on. But nowadays in popular culture the man in mid-life crisis is not a great artist groping his way to a sculpted creativity – whatever that is – but a deluded fool futilely trying to cheat time: dressing inappropriately, driving a sports car, a simmering mass of frustrated libido and lechery.

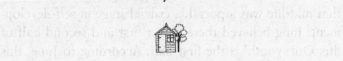

Autumn

Outside in the garden I start surveying the land. Drawing diagrams. Making plans. The leaves are beginning to glow gold. I take the dog out for pensive walks past hedgerows full of fruit: sloes, blackberries, crab apples, wild hops. Keats described autumn as a 'season of mists and mellow fruitfulness'. Others, however, are not so keen on the whole 'mellowing' thing. Woody Allen, for example. 'I don't respond well to mellow,' he says in *Annie Hall*. 'If I get too mellow, I ripen and then rot.'

I know what he means. I love autumn as a *season*, but not as a concept – you know, when people are described as being in the 'autumn' of their career, or even their lives. Their lives have blossomed, then bloomed – now things are starting to rot and drop off. As Macbeth said, 'my life is fallen into the sear, the yellow leaf'. To be fair, he was not in the most cheerily optimistic frame of mind at the time, having, after some very bad career advice from three witches, murdered several people and started seeing ghosts.

But even without all that Scottish blood and mayhem, the feeling of decline is common to middle age. We hear the whisper: it's all downhill from here. We're growing old. We grow old and mellow, we rot and die.

Well, you know, sod that. The more I began to examine this topic, and think about my own life in relation to it, the more determined I was to learn something about living. I don't know whether I'm in mid-life or beyond that, but I do know that I am not slowing down for anyone. And if I'm on the downslope, well, the thing about downslopes is this: they don't half allow you to build up a head of speed.

That's why Jung's insight is so important. Jung saw middle age not as a time of decline, but as a time of rebirth. Jung saw middle age as the time for individuation, the process by which people become whole. The psychologist and priest John Sanford explains individuation using the image of the oak tree. The oak tree is the individuated version of the acorn. The acorn grows into the oak because that's what it's intended to do. And no two oak trees are identical: 'When something individuates it becomes both a complete *and* unique expression of life.'[8]

11

As I looked around that autumn, I could see individuation starting all around me. That's the whole point of autumn. Fruit has to fall to the ground so that new, unique plants can grow. Jesus put it like this: 'Unless a grain of wheat falls into the earth and dies, it remains just a single grain; but if it dies, it bears much fruit' (John 12:24).

Autumn is a time to begin transformation and change.

And I was ready for change. Because I had already done the 'falling' bit.

2

INTO THE DARKNESS

The passport

Dante's poem *The Divine Comedy* is a three-part journey through hell, purgatory and finally heaven. It begins when the poet gets lost. 'Midway upon the journey of our life', he finds himself in a dark forest where 'the straightforward pathway had been lost'.[*]

Our mid-life journey starts with loss. And, for me, what was lost was a passport.

I was due to speak at a big event in France.[†] We were supposed to arrive on the Monday. On the Thursday before, I looked for my passport and couldn't find it anywhere. In a complete panic, I called the inappropriately named Passport and Identity Helpline who told me, unhelpfully, that yes, I would have to make a new application; no, I couldn't get an express passport issued; sorry,

---

[*] Dante was having a bit of a mid-life crisis himself. When he wrote *The Divine Comedy* his political career lay in ruins. The governing powers in Florence, his home city, had seized all his assets and sentenced him to death. He was exiled from the city of his birth, and never returned. It took until 2008 – nearly seven centuries after his death – for the city council of Florence to get around to rescinding his death sentence.

[†] Not in French. The only French words I know relate to food, wine and the occasional footballer.

it would take a week, and oh, by the way, if any passport office deigned to grant me an audience, it would be treated like a new application, so I would need to take with me my birth certificate, my parents' birth certificates, my grandparents' birth certificates, my special, magical name granted to me by the fairies, a four-leaf clover and £30,000 in used notes. Or something like that.

Now I realise, as I embark on this story, that this was not a big issue in the grand scheme of things. This was not some life-threatening disease. It wasn't a bereavement or a divorce or a redundancy or any of the usual life-shattering occurrences. But, for some reason, this event broke me.

All I could think of was that I was a complete failure. I was hopeless, helpless, I would let everyone down. Much to my own surprise, I ended up lying curled up on the bed, sobbing uncontrollably, convinced that my entire life was useless. For five days I was a shattered, shaky mass of anxiety. The Wife, full of wisdom, took me to the doctor, who – much to my surprise – used phrases like 'burnout' and 'a bit depressed' and prescribed me some tiny blue pills to help me sleep.

It all worked out OK, of course. Steve, the event manager, was gracious and wonderful and kind. I managed to get an appointment at the Passport Office in Peterborough, where a 14-year-old girl behind the counter pressed a button, ignored all the documentation I'd brought with me, looked at my new photo, said, 'Ooh, you look a bit older,' and issued me with a new passport. Eventually I made it to the event, one day late.

All things considered, it was a pretty minor occurrence. But it showed me the true state of myself. Just for a moment, the façade had slipped and revealed what my persona had kept hidden: deep feelings of failure and vulnerability. Someone in need of repair. I believe now that this collapse was a grace and a gift.

And it has stayed with me. Since then I have had a number of wobbles. I feel more prone to anxiety. In particular, the nights can sometimes be difficult. I wake in the darkness thinking about the future, or money, or health, or ... well, whatever.

And I have realised that I am far from alone. I've been amazed to find how many men have had similar experiences. Many have experienced what I did: moments of adversity that should pass but have somehow reduced them to rubble. For some these have developed, sadly, into full-blown depression. A great many men experience general feelings of anxiety, failure and loss.

Sometimes it really is the slightest thing that can set us off. One man I met – let's call him Steve – told me how he had returned from a long career serving as a missionary overseas. On the television he saw an advert for a DIY store. The adverts featured a series of men who were standing back admiring their handiwork and saying, 'I did that.' Suddenly this Steve bloke found himself in floods of tears: he believed that there was nothing in his life of which he could say, 'I did that.'

Of course he was wrong. But in his eyes, what he had achieved counted for nothing. I met another Steve at a church weekend at which I was speaking. He was a judge. He had reached the pinnacle of his career, had everything he was striving for. And at that point the drinking took over. Because he had spent his life striving to reach that position, only to find that when he got there, he felt as empty as ever.

Why is this? Why is it that so many men seem to have it all, and yet feel as though they have nothing? What is behind this question, 'Is that it?'

I have spent the past few years thinking about this, about the mid-life crisis in general and what it all means. And I have come to realise that these feelings are important. This stuff that we go through is not a blip. It's more than a bump in the road, after which we go on travelling in the same direction as before. No, these experiences *mean* something. These feelings of frustration or anger or failure or loss need to be listened to. If we pay attention to them, if we confront them and seek to understand them, we will find out what they really are.

They are a call. An invitation to new life.

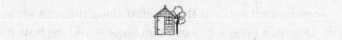

All at sea

Perhaps the greatest novel of mid-life crisis is, funnily enough, a children's book. Or that's how it's sold, anyway. It's called *Moominpappa at Sea*, written by Tove Jansson. The Swedish title of the book translates simply 'The Father and the Sea'. (If you don't know the Moomin books – what have you been doing with your life? Moomins are small troll-like creatures, and the series tells of their adventures in Moominland.) The books are wonderful, but as the series goes on they become more and more filled with themes of sadness and loss. Here's the opening of the book:

One afternoon at the end of August, Moominpappa was walking about in his garden feeling at a loss. He had no idea what to do with himself, because it seemed everything there was to be done had already been done or was being done by somebody else.[9]

Moominpappa has lost any sense of purpose. He feels he is no longer needed. And so he conceives of a grand project: he will take the family far out to sea, to live on an island. 'It's strange,' his wife, Moominmamma, muses. 'Strange that people can be sad, and even angry because life is too easy. But that's the way it is, I suppose. The only thing to do is to start life afresh.'[10]

And that is what I'm going to talk about in this book. I want to explore the idea that the experiences which so many men go through in mid-life are an invitation to a new start. But before we really get going, I think it's worth setting out my stall. Just so you know what's coming . . .

First, I want to examine the profound feelings of dislocation which afflict men in middle age. I think these feelings arise because we have been putting our faith in the wrong things. We have been worshipping the wrong gods.

Second, I want to look at how we fix this. Which, essentially, is doing all that 'Jung stuff': individuating. Growing into the person we were always meant to be. And this means understanding that God created us, and that it is our relationship with him which gives us all the status and security we need.

Finally, I want to explore how we experience that relationship and what it looks like in our lives. And basically, that means becoming a disciple – a trainee or an apprentice – of Jesus.

Here's the executive summary, for all you middle-aged executives: *The feelings men get in mid-life are a call to a deeper and more purposeful life. That life is found in a relationship with God, a relationship we enter into through learning from Jesus.*

I know, I know. Just when you thought this was going to be a light-hearted book about sheds, we're 'doing God'. Alarm bells are going off in your head right now. Maybe you were given this book by a well-meaning friend, relative or spouse. Maybe you thought it would be a book full of useful insights from neuroscience and psychology, and suddenly you are presented with a load of religious wibble. Maybe part of the problem is that you have tried the whole 'Jesus' thing and it has failed to live up to the advertising.

Let me reassure you a bit. I'm not asking you to sign your brain over to a cult. I'm not saying that if you 'give your life to Jesus' all your problems will magically disappear. And, actually, the Bible doesn't say that. I'm suggesting that through learning from Jesus and doing the stuff he did, we can find a new purpose and a deeper, richer, more contented life.

This may sound like airy-fairy religious nonsense, but, as we shall see, following Jesus is a demanding and challenging calling. And, what is more, as both Dante and Moominpappa have discovered, the way for many of us to enter this lies through a very dark night.

The dark night of the soul

Let's return for a moment to those feelings of abandonment. That 3 a.m. alarm call in your brain, where you wake and the Imax projector in your head starts to show a looping film of all the crap you have ever done. Those times when you are lost and stumbling and fearful and alone.

The medieval writers had a name for this kind of experience. They called it 'the dark night of the soul'.*

The phrase was coined by a man called John of Yepes, better known as John of the Cross. He was born in Castile, Spain, in 1542. After a harsh and difficult childhood, he became a monk. He became a prominent reformer within the Carmelite order, but his reforms made him enemies and he was kidnapped. He was beaten up, tried by a kind of ecclesiastical court and kept in solitary confinement in a dark, cramped, high-security cell. He was badly fed and not allowed to change his clothes. It was so cold that he developed frostbite in his toes. His captors would come and whisper lies through the door: 'No one cares about you', 'You have been forgotten', 'All your reforms have failed'. He was abandoned and alone.

In August 1588, weak and half-starved, he managed to escape from his cell with the help of a friendly prison guard. Using a rope fashioned out of his bedding, he lowered himself down a wall. The rope was too short and

---

* Not to be confused with the Dark Knight. That's Batman. Although you could say that dressing up in tight lycra, donning a cape and going out to pick a fight is classic mid-life behaviour.

he was forced to take a literal leap of faith, dropping into the blackness. Fortunately, he landed on an escarpment, climbed over a roof, made his way into the town and found refuge with some Carmelite nuns.

In the cell, he had begun to doubt himself and all that he had done. But he started to reflect on what he might learn from what he was going through. And in that darkness – *through* that darkness – he made sense of his life. Either in that cell, or a little after his escape, he wrote a poem, and he called it *Dark Night of the Soul*. John's phrase has come to be widely applied to those times when we feel our life is clouded and obscure, when we no longer feel God is with us, when we are lost and abandoned.

'The soul feels itself to be perishing and melting away,' he wrote, 'in the presence and sight of its miseries, by a cruel spiritual death, even as if it had been swallowed by a beast, and felt itself being devoured in the darkness of its belly.'[11]

It feels like death, but this dark night is a gateway to a new life of union with God. So John advised those in the darkness to

take comfort, to persevere in patience and to be in no wise afflicted. Let them trust in God, who abandons not those that seek him with a simple and right heart, and will not fail to give them what is needful for the road, until he bring them into the clear and pure light of love.[12]

Soul medicine

Modern science doesn't talk about the soul very much. It is a word that has been banished from psychiatry, psychotherapy and psychology, which is ironic since all of these take their names from *psyche* – the Greek word for 'soul'. (Psychotherapy is really soul medicine, therapy for the psyche.)

In my experience, most people acknowledge that there is something inside them, something which is uniquely *them*. The soul is very hard to define, but we know, instinctively, when something is wrong with it. We know when we are soul-sick. Someone who shows a lack of love or compassion is called soulless. If someone doesn't respond to something beautiful, we say to them, 'Oh, you have no soul.'

Throughout history, philosophers and sages have sought to take care of their souls. Perhaps the earliest example of this is an Egyptian book called *A Man in Dialogue with his 'Ba'*. 'Ba' means 'soul', and the work expresses the feelings of a depressed ancient Egyptian, who wonders why life seems so meaningless and whether he should just give up entirely.

'Behold, my name is detested,' he complains, 'more than the smell of vultures, on a summer's day when the sky is hot.' He goes on to say that his name is more detested, in fact, than smelly fish, smelly ducks, smelly fishermen, smelly crocodiles ... in short, life stinks. 'To whom can I speak today?' he asks. 'I am heavy-laden with trouble, through lack of an intimate friend.'[13] He is without a soulmate.

The soul – our inner being – is something that I would suggest matters to all of us. And, while I'm suggesting things left, right and centre, I'd also like to throw in the idea that, while John of the Cross's experience was somewhat unusual, it was far from being unique. Admittedly, not many of my readers will ever be put into solitary confinement by renegade monks, let alone escape to find refuge with Carmelite nuns, but those feelings of being shut in, closed off from the world, the feelings that the rest of the world has forgotten us, and more, that our life's work has come to nothing – well, *that* we can empathise with.

In fact, this experience is so fundamental to human nature that it forms the basis for nearly all our best stories.

In his seminal (and massive) book *The Seven Basic Plots*,[14] Christopher Booker outlines the core stories that we tell ourselves as human beings. Although he distinguishes seven styles, in many ways they all express a common, threefold progression. It begins with achievement. The hero sets out on a journey, or is given a task to perform or a problem to solve. At first things go well. He overcomes the early difficulties and progresses towards his goal. Then, inevitably, there comes a crisis, a moment when it all seems to have gone wrong. Hope dies. Possibilities fade. There is darkness and confusion. Finally there is a twist, a resolution. There is success. The hero defeats the monster, the exile returns home, the lovers are finally united.

We see this outline time and again in stories and plays and films. There is that moment of darkness, when everything is lost and there is no way out, and then – boom! – the plot twist, a sudden reversal.

Boom! Rocky Balboa switches to southpaw and knocks out Apollo Creed.

Boom! Jung emerges from the 'land of the dead' an individuated man.

Boom! The ugly duckling turns out to be a swan.

Boom! Moominpappa learns to let go of his need to control and brings his family back from the island.

Boom! John of Yepes escapes using a rope made of sheets.

Boom! Nick Page has a crappy few years but turns into a better person because of it.

Yep. We all have our own story, and all our stories are versions of the big story. Achievement, despair, resolution. Or, to put it another way, life, death and resurrection.

So let's look at one of those stories now. A story which, in my opinion, has much to tell us about mid-life, darkness, God and all that stuff.

3

THE WRESTLING MATCH

The twins

Genesis 32 contains one of the strangest stories in the Bible. It tells how the biblical patriarch Jacob – grandson of Abraham, father of Joseph (he of technicolour dreamcoat fame) – has a wrestling match with God.

The signs are there from the start. Jacob emerged from the womb holding onto the heel of his twin brother, Esau. And so he was named *Yaacov* – Jacob – which means 'grasper, supplanter'. He is grasping from the very first moment: it's in his nature.

That was how his life played out. His red-headed brother Esau was not one of life's deep thinkers. As a hunter, he was more of a shoot first, talk later kind of guy. And his sharper younger brother was able to run rings round him. First, Jacob tricked his brother out of his birthright. The eldest son had particular rights within ancient families: he was the leader of his brothers, and he was entitled to a double portion of any inheritance. But one day, Esau came back from the hunt to discover that Jacob was cooking a pot of something. And it smelt *great*.

'Give me some of that red stuff,' says Esau. So Jacob does, but in return he gets Esau to sign over his claim to the birthright. Esau – who is *starving*, really, completely famished, I'm going to die of hunger and I'm not even

25

joking – agrees. And so Jacob hands over the stew, and moves up the pecking order.

Round one to Jacob. Then, later, Jacob tricks Esau out of the blessing which Isaac intended to give to him. While Esau is out hunting for the 'blessing meal', Jacob – directed by his mother Rebekah – disguises himself as his elder brother, serves up a meal to his near-blind father, and receives the blessing instead.

Round two to Jacob. Jacob's character is clear. He is the trickster, the conman, astutely exploiting his opponent's weakness and winning through sheer duplicity. But there is a cost. This time Esau is not so laid back. When he finds out about the deception, he vows to kill Jacob.

So Jacob leaves home and heads north. And that's when he first encounters God. Outside the city of Luz, Jacob has a dream in which he sees angels going up and down some kind of stairway. And he hears from God, who promises that Jacob and his ancestors will own the land he is lying on and that the whole world will be blessed through his family. 'Know that I am with you and will keep you wherever you go,' says God, 'and will bring you back to this land; for I will not leave you until I have done what I have promised you' (Genesis 28:15).

When Jacob wakes, though, he sees it as a deal. He even tries to negotiate a food and clothing allowance: 'If God will be with me, and will keep me in this way that I go, and will give me bread to eat and clothing to wear, so that I come again to my father's house in peace, then the LORD shall be my God . . .' (Genesis 28:20-21).

When God made the same promise to Grandfather Abraham, the old man never tried to add anything on. He just stayed silent. Jacob, though, is a different kettle of fish. Or bowl of red stuff. He sees relationships as being like deals. God is a business partner. Still, heartened by this encounter, he goes on to his Uncle Laban's place. And there he meets three people: the girl of his dreams, the sister of the girl of his dreams, and their father, who is almost as tricky as Jacob. Almost.

Because here is where Jacob, slowly, starts to change. He falls in love with Rachel, Laban's daughter. He agrees to work for seven years for Laban, if he can marry Rachel. Laban agrees, but seven years later, on the day of the marriage, Laban does the old switcheroo and substitutes his other daughter, Leah, for Rachel. (The brides were heavily veiled. Think burka. Jacob could only see the eyes, and maybe not even those.) When Jacob finds out that he has been tricked, he's furious. He's maybe as furious as his brother Esau was when Jacob pulled the same kind of trick on him – not that Jacob seems to make that connection. Anyway, Laban promises him he can have Rachel as well, as long as he agrees to work for another seven years. So that's what Jacob does.

And he gets his revenge. Over the next decade and a half or so Jacob works off his 'debt' and builds up his own flock. He cunningly makes himself rich through a strange kind of selective breeding programme which means that, despite his uncle's attempts to fool him, Jacob's flocks are the strongest, the best bred and the most numerous.

By now, though, the relationship between the two has soured. So, once again, Jacob flees, although not without taking with him as much as he can get away with.

And so we come to the wrestling match.

'A man wrestled with him . . .'

By now, we know what we need to know about Jacob. He's the archetypal over-achiever, the supplanter, the master of sharp practice. Whatever happens, Jacob comes out on top. He's the type of person who could follow you into a revolving door and somehow come out in front.

But now Jacob is in trouble. He can't return to Laban. Those bridges have been well and truly burned. Then he hears that Esau is on his way to meet him with a force of four hundred men. So he can't go back, he's terrified of going forward and, for the first time in his life, he can't think of any way to get out of this.

He has to have a plan. First thing: damage limitation. He splits his camp into two companies, thinking that if Esau butchers one, then the other will escape. But it's not enough. He *knows* it's not enough.

So Jacob does something that we have not seen him do before. For the first time in this story, Jacob prays. 'I am not worthy of the least of all the steadfast love and all the faithfulness that you have shown to your serv-ant . . . Deliver me, please, from the hand of my brother, from the hand of Esau, for I am afraid of him' (Genesis 32:10-11). Before, it's been God who has spoken to Jacob, through dreams, and dreams are a passive, one-way communication. Now Jacob speaks back. He needs to talk to God. He wants rescue. He wants salvation.

After the prayer, he comes up with a new plan: he starts sending advance parties ahead with gifts of camels and cows and sheep and goats to appease his red-haired, hot-headed brother. So he sends his wives and children, his servants, his livestock on ahead – everything, all the booty of his duplicitous years. He's left with nothing and nobody. He is utterly alone. And then you get this line: 'Jacob was left alone; and a man wrestled with him until daybreak' (Genesis 32:24).

Here's the Bible account:

> The same night he got up and took his two wives, his two maids, and his eleven children, and crossed the ford of the Jabbok. He took them and sent them across the stream, and likewise everything that he had. Jacob was left alone; and a man wrestled with him until daybreak. When the man saw that he did not prevail against Jacob, he struck him on the hip socket; and Jacob's hip was put out of joint as he wrestled with him.
>
> Then he said, 'Let me go, for the day is breaking.' But Jacob said, 'I will not let you go, unless you bless me.' So he said to him, 'What is your name?' And he said, 'Jacob.'
>
> Then the man said, 'You shall no longer be called Jacob, but Israel, for you have striven with God and with humans, and have prevailed.' Then Jacob asked him, 'Please tell me your name.' But he said, 'Why is it that you ask my name?' And there he blessed him. (Genesis 32:22-29)

So, a fight, and a renaming. Jacob is given the name Israel. He names the site Peniel, which means 'face of God'. 'I have seen God face to face,' he says, 'and yet my life is preserved.' And, as the sun rises, he limps off to see his brother Esau, where he finds that all is well. Esau is prosperous and contented and has forgiven the events of twenty years before.

But Jacob is clearly changed by this encounter. He is wounded, and he is renamed.

That's the story, anyway. Of course, there are many questions. Who is the man? Did God really fight with Jacob? If it was God, why did he ask Jacob his name – surely he knew? And if he could just dislocate Jacob's hip in a moment like that, why didn't he do so earlier? Why does he give Jacob a new name anyway?

What on earth is this all about?

I'll come back to those questions in due course. But for now the key thing to note is that Jacob had reached a point where everything that he had struggled to achieve in his life was of no help to him. At that point, in the middle of the night, he was alone, facing failure and fear and the humiliating realisation that there was no way he could fix this. He had nothing to bargain with, he could no longer cut a deal with God.

In many ways, by this point Jacob was a success. Anyone looking at him from a distance would have thought him to be flourishing. He had wives, children, servants, flocks. But the reality was different. He was older now. He was scared. And he was suddenly faced with something over which he had no control and through which no trickery would guide him.

This is the original 'dark night'. This was the lowest point in his life. And that was exactly the point when he had his deepest encounter with God.

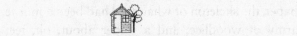

Clearing out

A few days after my vision, we emptied the old shed. The costumes from decades of The Wife's theatre projects went upstairs into the loft. Behind them I discovered a museum of abandoned projects, a forgotten land of rubbish. Tins of paint going back many decades. Fittings for power tools that I no longer owned. Old user manuals. Computer cables, for computers which had long since departed the Page household. Electrical plugs from the years when electrical equipment didn't come with a plug on it. Above all, all the stuff I'd gathered 'in case it came in useful'.

I had underestimated the state of the shed.

From the outside it didn't look that bad. But inside it was a complete mess.

The roof was rotten, as were some parts of the walls. The floor, though sound enough, was not what you'd call in the prime of life. Where the water had come through the roof in the far corner, it had dripped down onto a set of steel shelves. The bottom shelves were so rusty that, as I tried to pick them up, they crumbled, with an acrid smell. Strange how such a strong material could be turned to dust by nothing but rain water.

I moved an old sideboard which had served as a bench. The first time it had been moved in about fifteen years.

Behind it were unimaginable horrors, including but not limited to cobwebs, rotted rags, some bits of unidentifiable paper, the skeleton of what once had been a mouse, a small army of woodlice, and a spider about, oh, feet long. I bravely fought off the spider, with the aid of a broom, and disposed of the remains of the mouse. There was ivy growing through the wall. I thought about pulling it out, but had a suspicion it was the only thing holding the wall up.

Moving all the contents meant some heavy lifting and the next day my back was playing up. Curious phrase. We talk about backs 'playing up' as if they were teenagers, moaning adolescents, but the effect of backs playing up is to make you very old, very quickly. A bad back turns you instantly into an old man. Everything becomes slower, more careful. Getting out of bed is like stop-motion animation. Putting your socks on is like trying to get into a particularly difficult yoga position.

Eventually I made it to the bathroom and looked at the stranger in the mirror. I wonder if Jacob looked at himself the same way. Was the river water still enough for him to look at his own face? Did he see a stranger submerged in the depths?

There were two men in the mirror in front of me. One of them was balding, slightly weatherbeaten. But inside I could see another man, about twenty-four years old, young, virile; still capable, he thinks, of achieving great things. Inside every middle-aged man is a young man struggling to grow up.

Growing older

Satchel Paige, who was a well-known baseball pitcher in the US, once asked a very important question: 'How old would you be if you didn't know how old you was?'[15] Our internal clock runs at a different speed to the real world. On the eve of her fiftieth birthday, and presumably sitting in her shed, Virginia Woolf wrote, 'I sometimes feel that I have lived 250 years already, and sometimes that I am the youngest person on the omnibus.'[16] We contain, inside of us, all the time periods we have lived through, all the selves we have been, and, indeed, all the selves we still hope to be. This is why physical ageing is such a surprise for us: inside, we simply do not feel that old.

It's a shock to see ourselves growing older. I saw a video of myself, taken recently on a trip to Africa, and I genuinely didn't recognise the figure. I had let my beard grow long for the trip, under the mistaken belief that a longer beard guarantees respect. I looked like one of the lesser patriarchs in Genesis, although if I'd gone to the Tower of Babel I'd never have made it up the stairs.

I have this old person's thing now. I am unable to make any upward or downward movement without some accompanying noise. I sit down and grunt. I bend over to pick something up and grunt. It doesn't matter how heavy the object is: I could be picking up a feather, I still grunt. I don't know why I do this, or when it started. But it's instinctive.

Muscles ache. Bones creak. Eyesight declines. I can no

longer grow hair on my head, but I can't stop it growing out of my ears. I get tired more quickly. It hits 8 p.m. and I start to think about going to bed. I am getting old. And though this is a perfectly natural, ordinary process, it's also really, really annoying.

All organisms age. Well, amoebas don't: an old amoeba looks exactly the same as a young one, but amoebas use asexual reproduction and have no social life to speak of. Apparently sex and death go hand in hand. You can't have one without the other, otherwise the planet would be even more crowded than it is.

Scientists are frustrated on the issue of ageing, because they don't really know why it happens. Some believe it's evolutionary: essentially we age and die so that a new, improved generation might come along and replace us. I think you can disprove this theory pretty quickly by looking at the young people in *Made in Chelsea*. If that's an improvement, I'm an amoeba.[17]

Animals do seem to have built-in ageing systems, but these vary greatly even within species. One species of mollusc can live four hundred times longer than another closely related and very similar species. Speed of life seems to have something to do with it: tortoises live a lot longer than cheetahs. This is my argument for lounging on my sofa most Saturday afternoons: I am merely improving my longevity.

But despite my best efforts not to move at any speed faster than a tortoise, I cannot cheat my biology. What happens to us in middle age is that certain biological processes kick in, and no amount of anti-ageing product is going to make any difference.

Muscle turns to fat and gravitates to the waist, leading

to the infamous middle-aged spread. And because, by middle age, most of us have shifted all the heavy lifting and active jobs onto younger idiots and spend our time behind a desk trying to look busy, we don't do enough physical exercise to get rid of it easily.

Worse, as the fat piles on, the skin is less able to hold it all in. The skin is made up of two main bits. On the top is the epidermis, the waterproof bit. Over time this becomes thinner and more translucent. I remember, when I was young, looking at the skin on the back of my grandmother's hands: it was wrinkled like tissue paper.

Below the epidermis is the dermis, a tougher layer full of protein fibres called collagen and elastin. These fibres give the skin its elasticity, which means that when you rise from your seat, for example, your skin snaps back into place instead of retaining a nasty crease mark across the middle. But collagen and elastin also deteriorate over time. Basically, the elastic in our body wears out, like a tired old pair of underpants. As we get older, things stop pinging back into place and just stay where they were put. So eyelids droop, cheeks sag. The whole effect can be summed up in one hideous word: moob. We are all at the mercy of gravity.

Nothing will stop us ageing. (Well, there is one thing that stops it, but most of us don't want that.) Anti-ageing creams are pretty much smoke and mirrors. Botox only makes it look as though someone has over-inflated your forehead.

So much for the exterior. Inside things are different as well. Our senses are not as sharp. Many cognition tests show a slowing down of processing speed in our brains. We cannot see or hear as well as we used to. Generally, I need to have a teenager permanently on hand in order to read the small print on instructions. We don't even smell as acutely as before.

Whatever your feelings about middle age, this one fact is universal: we are all growing older. This part of the process is completely unavoidable. 'Things fall apart', as Yeats so cheerily put it.

Man, I need a drink.

OK. So that's the position. But it's not as grim as it seems. Those cognition tests I just mentioned, for example: they are all about speed. And, as any middle-aged man will tell you, speed is over-rated. Tests which involve rapid recognition or response will naturally be more suited to younger people because (a) they don't like to take the time to do things properly, and (b) 'not thinking things through' comes naturally to them.

Once you take the need for speed out of the equation, you find a different picture. Many other types of cognitive tests, involving such things as verbal skills, spatial perception, mathematics, reasoning and planning, show that our brains are actually *better* in middle age. Mathematical skills peak around 40, verbal skills around 60.

Middle-aged brains are clever in a different way. First, there is the experience factor – older people simply *know* more than younger people. We know how to do things right, because we have learnt from a lifetime of doing things wrong. We know what corners can be cut.

I used to play five-a-side football with other members of my church, among whom were several very good and very fast teenagers. But they didn't have what I had, i.e., years of knowing how to crush the spirit of anyone younger, fitter and better looking than me. And so I could hold my own against them (a bit). And, as I helped them back to their feet after mashing them brutally against the wall, I would remind them of a very important life lesson: 'old age and cunning will always beat youth and talent'.

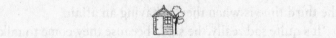

Shedding light

On the coldest day of the year, my mate Steve came to help me put some new windows in the shed. The existing windows – and I use the word loosely – consisted of two small pieces of grimy plastic and a piece of cracked glass held in place by an old rusty nail. They managed to radically rewrite the whole concept of windows by simultaneously keeping the light out while letting the cold air in. In defiance of all the laws of thermodynamics, it was actually colder inside the shed than outdoors.

Anyway, I had scavenged a set of double-glazed windows from a skip down the road, so we set about replacing them. It was an act which required precise, careful measurement and cutting. So naturally we just went at it like madmen, flailing away with the electric saw and filling the gaps with slim strips of spare softwood.

Surprisingly, it worked, and by the end of the day the old, dark shed was flooded with light. Or would have been had it not been (a) January and (b) 5 p.m. We sat in the gloom sipping our coffee.

Steve is a doctor. And he told me of his experiences in treating Men Of A Certain Age.

'Typically, I see men at three times in their life,' he said.

'The first time is at their first antenatal appointment – and then you never see them again at any subsequent antenatal appointment. The second time is after the baby is born, at the six-week check-up.' He sipped his coffee. 'And then the third time is when they're having an affair.'

'It's quite sad really,' he said, 'because they come to talk to me as their doctor about stuff that really is to do with them not having their life sorted out. It's that thing you talk about. They've climbed up the hill only to look across and realise they're on the wrong mountain. So they get a real sense of dislocation and disorientation.'

'How does that manifest itself?' I asked.

'You get two sorts of syndromes. One is the psychological problems like insomnia, anxiety, stress, depression. Or addictions, like alcohol, drugs, exercise.'

'Exercise?'

'I get a lot of middle-age injuries. It's kind of a recognised phenomenon in the orthopaedic world. Forty-year-old men are getting cruciate ligament injuries that 20-year-old footballers get. But of course the difference is that they don't heal as quickly. And we get more early presentations of osteoarthritis because they are basically over-using their joints.'

'And the other manifestation?'

'What we call somatisation. Psychological problems presenting as physical problems. So people come in with headaches. And they all get chest pain. You can't take the risk that they *haven't* got heart problems, because they're in the at-risk group. You know, the archetypal businessman sat in his convertible Mercedes drives around and starts to get chest pain – you're going to be a brave man to say, "Aha – I think it's your mid-life crisis." So you investigate. You do your ECGs and blood tests and you find something that's not 100 per cent as it should be on the test, which is very common. Then people latch on to that and you get into a whole cycle of medicalising what is primarily a social or psychosocial problem.

'The last thing they want to hear is that there's something psychologically wrong with them: they want a quick fix. But they have to address what the problem is and find the solution. If you hide behind medication either as an excuse or a sticking plaster, you're not really addressing the key turmoil that's going on in the mind.'

My conversation with Steve confirmed what I had come to believe: that it is too easy to dismiss the problems of middle age as being merely about 'getting older'. Psychologically, of course, that has an effect. But even though our bodies are ageing, that doesn't mean we are on an inexorable downhill path. There are plenty of years and opportunities ahead. I don't think that, in the end, it is the mere fact of growing older physically which makes men experience these 'dark night' feelings of middle age. I think it is something more fundamental.

It is not so much the failure of their bodies; it is the failure of their gods.

4

THE GODS WHO FAILED

The wrong gods

Let me tell you about an Egyptian god. He was, in fact, a god of salvation – popularly known as the 'saviour' – a god that the Egyptians looked to in order to save them from illness, misfortune or danger. He never had any temples or any kind of formal cult; he was very much a domestic god. And his name was, of course, Shed.

Shed worship seems to have arisen as a popular response to attempts by an emperor called Akhenaten to get rid of the ancient religion of Egypt. Ordinary people didn't like the newfangled ideas that Akhenaten was bringing in. So they created Shed – a god who, insofar as he appeared anywhere, was shown vanquishing their enemies: serpents, scorpions, crocodiles. Maybe, even, very large spiders.

Shed, therefore, was a kind of Egyptian anti-authority deity, a helper for ordinary people. As time went on, his abilities expanded. He was credited with being able to save a person from the underworld, or lengthen the days of someone's life.

Shed, of course, is long gone. But I like to think that today he does have some temples. They are found in gardens, backyards, allotments, little anti-authoritarian

41

places of protection offering sanctuary and shelter when help isn't coming from anywhere else.*

After all, everyone needs a saviour. Especially when society can't provide one.

In the last week of his life, Jesus was in the temple when he was asked a question by a scribe – a kind of local religious official. 'Which commandment is the first of all?' asked the scribe. This was a man whose job was to help people obey God's instructions, to tell them, essentially, how to live. But there were more than six hundred commandments or instructions in the Jewish code, so if you could only do one thing, what would it be? Jesus replied with two quotes from the books of the law:

> 'The first is, "Hear, O Israel: the Lord our God, the Lord is one; you shall love the Lord your God with all your heart, and with all your soul, and with all your mind, and with all your strength." The second is this, "You shall love your neighbour as yourself." There is no other commandment greater than these.' (Mark 12:29-31)

For Jesus, it all comes down to what you love and what – or who – you worship.

One of the most important themes in the Bible is idolatry – the worship of false gods. The reason is simple: what you worship defines your life. We all worship something, or someone. In Jesus' day most cities in the Roman Empire

---

* The iconography of Shed usually shows him as a child or young man, most often with a shaved head and wearing a kilt. Personally I'm going to claim that he was actually a naturally bald middle-aged bloke who just had babyish features.

were full of temples dedicated to the gods. You could not walk down a street or even enter a home without encountering a god of some sort. Today we like to imagine that we are above such things, but we have gods and temples just the same. A nation's gods are always indicated by their biggest buildings. It used to be churches, now it's office blocks and banks and luxury high-rise apartments. The skyline of London is a tribute to the gods of the city: money, status, luxury and power.

It is very easy to create a god. All you do is put something on a pedestal and expect miracles out of it. And our basic problem in mid-life is that this is when we come to realise that our gods have failed us. This is why feelings of disappointment and failure are so often associated with middle age. It's not that *we* have actually failed – at least not in the ways that we think. It is our gods that have failed us. We trusted them. We did as we were told. We made all the proper sacrifices.

But they turned out to be the wrong gods.

What would an ancient Greek make, I wonder, of our cities and temples and gods?

Let us, for a moment, look at the pantheon of gods in this kingdom of middle age. Let us name and shame the gods who failed.

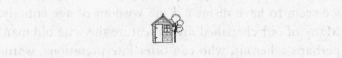

God #1: Lycra, the god of youth

Sub-deities: Toupée, god of hair restoration; Nipantuck, god of cosmetic surgery; Mutton, god of slightly-too-tight denim; Triathlon, god of extreme sports.

Many cities in the empire have shrines to Lycra. The citizens call them 'gyms'. I believe this is derived from our gymnasia. Of course, in our day, gymnasia were temples not only of the body but of the mind, with libraries and lecture halls. But in this world, the emphasis is on the body and the outward appearance. The god demands from his people regular sacrifices in the form of physical activity. His adherents are daily to be found running along the streets. His more dedicated worshippers undergo extreme physical torment – running many miles, or swimming across lakes in order to please him. The icons of Lycra show him as male or female, but always young, strong, beautiful and with what his worshippers call 'a six-pack'.

When I was growing up, prime ministers and presidents were *supposed* to be old. It granted them wisdom and experience. That's why they were *elder* statesmen. Previous generations knew what a rich resource wisdom was. Age, of course, doesn't grant you wisdom automatically. I have met many very old, very unwise people. But we seem to have dismissed the wisdom of age entirely. Many of our cherished myths feature the wise old man, perhaps a hermit, who can offer interpretations, warnings and advice for the younger hero. In the story of Odysseus, for example, during the *nekyia*, the trip to the land of the dead, he meets the wise old man Teiresias who tells him what lies in the future, and what more Odysseus has to do to complete his journey.

Now society is in the grip of a cult of youth. We are neophiliacs, desperate for the new and the young. In a way, it's our fault: after all, we were the baby boomers, the ones who decided that everyone old was 'square'. But we didn't really know what we were saying. The Who sang, 'hope I die before I get old' – now Roger Daltrey is over 70, and we're just confused.

We don't believe in the wise old man, but the old fogey. Ever since Mr and Mrs Blair had a baby in Downing Street, politicians have been desperate to appear younger and full of street cred. (Some might say we could have done with a few older and wiser heads in power: maybe then we wouldn't have started so many wars.)

It's all part of a youth cult that is driven by a horror of old age. It's all about being – or pretending to be – young.

At the same time there is little discussion of growing older positively. There is a lot of stuff about how to cheat old age. But there is not much mature thought on how to enjoy its benefits – and even embrace the advantages it can bring. Instead all we get are *Daily Express* front-page scare stories: Alzheimer's, dementia, poverty. Our view of ageing is coloured by fear. We are petrified of being petrified.

Generally, men react to growing older in two main ways: defiance and denial.

Defiance first. These are the MAMILs – middle-aged men in Lycra. *Come on ageing – do your worst. I'm not over the hill yet. Fetch me the unsuitably tight Lycra, I'm off to take up the triathlon.*

Let's take one such MAMIL. Steve runs. He cycles. He swims. Sometimes he does all three in one day, in the triathlon. He has run not one, but two marathons. He is thinking of going on to do even more extreme challenges: running up mountains, crossing deserts. Something called the 'Iron Man' challenge. 'I want to prove that I can still do it,' he tells me. 'You know I'm fitter than the guys half my age.'

He's certainly fitter than me, but I get the feeling with Steve that there is more to it than that. I notice a marked tendency among Men Of A Certain Age to take things to extremes, to push themselves further and further. Nothing wrong with that, I suppose. I am full of admiration for friends who have run a marathon and full of envy of those who can easily cycle a hundred miles and then hop up a nearby mountain. But it does seem from my vantage point (i.e. sitting on a chair in the pub) that they are trying to prove something.*

On the whole, the desire to push the boundaries of physical achievement is a good thing. It gives you a sense of purpose. But other men take up running in a non-literal sense: instead of running their way *through* middle age, they run *away* from it.

This is the denial response. Men start to dress younger. The jeans grow tighter. A tattoo appears. Maybe even an ill-advised ponytail. At the extreme is the ageing celebrity with the unnaturally black hair and plastic-smooth

---

* Actually I do keep reasonably fit. I play squash once a week, which leaves me the colour of a freshly boiled lobster and wheezing like a geriatric goat. Fortunately my squash partner is a GP so he can administer CPR when needed.

botoxed skin, spray-tanned the colour of a tangerine, a bottle-blonde trophy-bride on his arm.

It's a good thing that older people are fitter, healthier, more active, generally a lot trendier than they were when I was growing up. As sociologist Andrew Blaikie wrote, 'Older citizens are encouraged not just to dress "young" and look youthful, but to exercise, have sex, diet, take holidays, and socialise in ways indistinguishable from those of their children's generation.'[18]

It's good to be able to dress however we want – but the question is whether we are feeling free in choosing our clothes, or driven to put on a costume. The risk is that we are trying to play the part of a younger man. Our appearance unintentionally reveals our inner life. My father, for example, started wearing a toupée and driving a sports car. It may have concealed his baldness, but it certainly revealed his insecurities. A lot of the show of the mid-life crisis is a man's way of trying to demonstrate that he's still 'got it'.

For some people, the desire to look young really comes out of a fear of maturity and responsibility. Far worse than the man who dresses ridiculously young is the man who *acts* ridiculously young. The eternal boy, the middle-aged adolescent, desperately trying to remain the centre of their own universe. It's a middle-aged adolescence: what Gail Sheehy calls 'middlescence'. One definition of the 'middlescent' is 'middle-aged but exhibiting behaviour or having interests more like an adolescent, esp. in choice of activities and fashion'.[19]

If we make a god of youth, then we are bound to fall short. No god is more certain to let us down in the end. Growing older doesn't mean having to give up youthful activities. Or – heaven forbid – youthful attitudes. But there's a difference between being childlike and being child-ish. None of us has a choice over whether or not to grow old. But we do have a choice as to whether we grow up.

God #2: Dosh, the god of wealth and possessions

Sub-deities: Argos, god of cheap consumer goods; Ferrari, god of fast cars; Saga, god of a comfortable retirement.

The temples of Dosh are the biggest and most glorious in the empire. Some of them are called 'banks', others are called 'shops'. In the main cities of the empire, they dominate the skyline. Dosh – or Mammon, to give him his ancient name – is an angry and demand-ing god, who seems determined to instil anxiety among his followers. Worshippers are constantly warned about the effects of inadequate reverence on growth forecasts. The high priests of this cult are called economists and, though they claim to know the future, they are none-theless constantly surprised by events. The gods send messages to their followers in what are known as adverts.

Let me tell you about my colleague Steve. I could see that Steve was becoming more and more unhappy at his work. He felt that no one was listening to him. He felt unappre-ciated. A lovely man, but you could tell that he was simmering with discontent. He got embroiled in a dispute over some kind of management decision – I never did work out what it was.

'How are you?' I asked him one day.

He grinned sheepishly. 'I did something I've never done

before over the weekend,' he said. 'I did some retail therapy.'

'Really? What did you buy?'

'A Porsche.'

'Steve,' I said to him. 'You do realise that all that will happen is that you'll just be unhappy at a higher speed.'

He shrugged. 'I'm not sure really why I did it,' he said.

But I knew why he did it. He did it because he was sad. And he thought that buying something extravagant was the way to cure his sadness.

Men are acquisitive. It's often said that men don't like shopping, but I don't think that's really true. What we don't like are shops. Most men are notorious collectors and hoarders. For example, I still have my vinyl record collection – and I still add to it, from time to time. I have thousands of books. I have boxes and boxes of comics. I am a stationery hoarder – I have more pens and note-books than I know what to do with. Some of my notebooks are so beautiful that I have never dared to write in them: I simply don't have thoughts worthy of those books. I could go on. I am obsessed with bags; I have a bag for everything and my life is perhaps best understood as a quest to find the perfect bag.

One of my absolute favourite books is a book called *Cool Tools*, which not only lists thousands of gadgets, tools, books, clothes and other items, but also why they are so good. And this is great, because men especially like buying stuff if it requires research. Because then it's not just a purchase, it's a task. And not only do we buy the object we need – a computer, a bag, a new pair of shoes – but we also have all the arguments ready over why our choice is the best. We can then get into debates online with complete strangers over why their choice of computer/bag/shoes was the wrong one. We are validated by our purchases.

And buying stuff gives us hope. I always think that the next thing will be The One, the single object which will change my life. The next pen I buy will be the one pen I need for the rest of my life. The next car I get will solve everything. We are buying dreams.

Car sellers understand this. Cars are sold on emotion. When was the last time you saw a car advert that told you anything about engineering or specifications? Instead, nearly all car adverts show you a car on an empty, winding road – usually in Scotland, or somewhere similarly mountainous and beautiful – with the vehicle moving like a sleek animal through the landscape. They are not selling you the car, they are selling you freedom. Freedom, but with monthly payments. The same thinking lies behind celebrity endorsements. We are not being sold a product, but the dream of celebrity. We think that buying a pair of Calvin Klein underpants will make us look like David Beckham looks on the posters. The truth is, it's not the underpants that make him look like that: it's a heady mixture of training, genetics and Photoshop. Even David Beckham doesn't really look like he does on the ads.

Our need to possess reveals an emptiness inside us. There is nothing wrong with buying things. The problem is that we expect it to bring us happiness.

At its worst, the need to possess is an addiction. And, as with all addictions, we become habituated to the drug; we need larger and larger doses from our dealer in order to feel anything. *Time was when I could get high on a dose of Ford; now I really need to score a BMW, or maybe some Mercedes, if you've got the stuff*. Our lives become distorted, bent towards the accumulation of money or possessions.

Jacob was a man whose entire life was built around acquiring stuff – birthrights, blessings, livestock, tents, wives, children, whatever he could get his hands on. And still he ended up wrestling with God in the dark, just like everyone. It is no coincidence that Jacob sent all his possessions on ahead of him. His dark night occurs when he has nothing around him at all. And it is noticeable that, after his fight with the Almighty, his acquisitiveness is gone. When he finally meets Esau, his estranged brother tries to return all the presents Jacob has sent him. But Jacob insists: 'God has dealt graciously with me . . . I have everything I want' (Genesis 33:11).

At its root, all of this is about wealth. Wealth can be in the form of cash in the bank, or bricks and mortar, or a Porsche. Now, I have been poor and I have been slightly less poor. And out of these two choices, I definitely prefer the second one. So I'm not knocking money, but money doesn't really have that much effect on happiness. There is clear empirical evidence to show that for most people in the West, our happiness quotient has not increased since 1950. In the US, although standards of living have almost doubled since the 1950s, people are no happier. In the UK, surveys show that happiness has been static since 1975.[20]

Wealth can increase happiness, but generally that is when it lifts people out of poverty. Surveys show that in countries where the average income is above $20,000, any additional income is not associated with extra happiness.[21] One explanation given is that any extra happiness brought by an increased standard of living has been cancelled out because our social relationships are correspondingly poorer.[22] Poor areas often have a stronger sense of solidarity and community.

And the ladder of possessiveness has no end. There is always something bigger and better to buy. There is always a new model. The first person in the street to get a BMW might feel good. But if everyone in the street has one, any thrill disappears.

The evidence is clear. This money-obsessed society has failed to deliver to us the one thing which we all need: happiness. Yet still the worship of money is taken for granted in our society. Economic growth is the be-all and end-all. News readers breathlessly deliver the latest stock market figures as if they were messages from the gods. *The FTSE has risen by 30 points. The god must be pleased with us!* It is taken for granted that this god has to be worshipped at all costs and any questioning of this assumption is greeted with a patronising smile, as if we don't understand, or don't live in the real world. *Don't anger the god,* we're told. *If we don't let money do what it wants, the financial temples might move elsewhere.*

It's not just that we have created false gods; we have created false gods who are 'too big to fail'.

Gods #3 and #4: The twins: Exhaustus, god of work, and Kudos, god of status

Sub-deities: Bonus, god of success; Agenda, god of meetings; Sardine, god of commuting.

The worshippers of Exhaustus and Kudos are easily identified by their long worship services – typically from early in the morning until early evening, with worship often continuing on the train home and even at weekends. Some of their worship services are in small temples known as 'meeting rooms', where adherents will sit for hours chanting their 'buzzwords' and meditating – or, as they call it, 'blue-sky thinking'. The temples of their gods are many and varied, but can be identified by the many small sacrificial altars inside, known as cubicles, which contain the screens through which worshippers commune with their god. Worshippers of Exhaustus live in fear of being cast out of his presence in the festival of sacrifice they call The Great Downsizing.

There's a wonderful Frank Cotham cartoon from the *New Yorker* magazine. Two American businessmen are sitting at a bar, nursing their bourbons. 'I usually wake up screaming at six-thirty,' says one, 'and I'm in the office at nine.'

Never mind the nightmares, you have to get the paperwork done.

Our work is a demanding god, and we serve it faithfully. According to one survey, British workers work 26 million extra hours in the workplace each day. Nearly 80 per cent of these hours are unpaid, meaning workers are providing around £225 million worth of 'free' hours each day for employers. Stress has become the most common cause of long-term sickness absence for both manual and non-manual employees. Nearly one in five workers say they have called in sick because of stress, but the vast majority of these – 93 per cent – lied to their boss about the real reason for not turning up.[23]

Our work is a major cause of anxiety and dissatisfaction. It's not only the money, it's also the power, the influence, the lure of the organisational chart. Every company has one, and we all know that the point in life is to move yourself up, level by level. Even when you don't want to.

I was recently chatting to a guy at a party. Can't remember his name, but it was probably Steve. He had just applied for a promotion.

'Well, I hope you get the job,' I said.

He laughed. 'I don't want it.'

'Why did you apply for it?'

'Because you have to,' he said. 'They expect you to apply for promotion. Else they don't think you're taking your career seriously.'

'What will you do if you get the job?' I asked.

He shook his head. 'I don't know. I really don't know.'

Steve was doing what the god of work required. We are told to find a job, work long hours, seek promotion and climb the ladder. Then we will get our prize. But the experience of many men in middle age is that they reach the top of the career ladder, only to find that the ladder was leaning against the wrong wall. There is no lonelier moment than when you get what you thought would bring you happiness, only to realise that it doesn't live up to your dreams.

The god of work is, for many men, a brutal deity. It encourages us to see ourselves entirely through its lens, so much so that many men define themselves by their jobs. Their definition of themselves as a success or a failure is based entirely on position: pay, promotion, achievements. Then one day they start to see signs of the god's displeasure. They are passed over for promotion, or shunted into a dead-end job. Where once their opinions and expertise were valued, now they are ignored, while a group of chinless wonders, the ink still dry on their management school MBAs, move into their territory. Perhaps most devastating, one day the god discards them completely. They are called into the manager's office, their only crime that they are more experienced than those around them, with longer service and commensurately higher pay. Success turns to failure in a moment. No wonder William James talked of 'the bitch goddess: Success'.[24]

Unemployment is a major factor in mid-life depression. But research shows that when people become unemployed, their happiness falls more because of their loss of purpose and status, than because they have lost income.

We are cannibalised by our careers. They eat away at our lives. Again, the issue is not the thing itself – we *need* to work. A productive, meaningful job is something which brings fulfilment. But if we place our job on a pedestal we will be ruined in the end.

Status matters. Everyone needs to feel valued. Some scientists experimented on groups of monkeys, manipulating a monkey's status by moving him from one group to another or rewarding him with food and special treatment. In each situation, the monkey's level of seroto-nin – the neurotransmitter associated with feeling good – rose. The higher the monkey's position in the hier-archy, the better the monkey felt. Or take another group of primitive primates: British civil servants. Those of higher rank have been shown to secrete lower average levels of cortisol, a stress-related hormone. They also live longer.[25]

Status is often closely linked with our work, but it can come from other areas of achievement as well. Some people try to gain status through their possessions and lifestyle, leading to high levels of debt in order to main-tain the life they think is expected of them. Others seek success – and therefore status – through mastering a hobby or a sport. Some seek a social position: magistrate, chair of various committees.

Others find status through their families. Some men find it difficult to adapt to the changing roles of father-hood. When they were little, our children relied on us for everything. But as they get older, the role changes. We become a taxi service, a handyman, a chef – or a cash-dispenser, a kind of human ATM. But we are no longer the god-like father figure that we once were when they were, oh, say, 6. They don't really need *us*, or so it seems.

One of the commonest feelings accompanying middle age is that of being useless, forgotten, taken for granted, sidelined.

'Nobody at home listens to me any more,' complained Steve. 'I used to be the life and soul of the party. Everyone else finds me funny, why don't they?'

I had been friends with Steve and his wife – Mrs

Steve – for a long time. Recently Steve had become hard to live with. Grumpy, irascible. Demanding. Work was difficult. He'd had to retrain; there were all kinds of management changes. He would arrive home at night looking to relax, only to find that everyone had their own agenda, and feel as though no one was taking any notice of him.

'No one appreciates me,' he said.

He was certainly deeply unhappy. As we supped our pints, he admitted to me that there was another woman: someone who, he said, really appreciated him. Who laughed at his jokes and gave him the attention he craved.

A number of questions flashed through my mind. Mainly, I was wondering why he felt the need to be the centre of attention. You expect that in an 8-year-old, not in someone in their late forties.

'Steve,' I said, 'you're not a child any more.'

'I know,' he said. 'But I just need to feel as though I matter. It feels like I'm invisible.'

Steve spent his time watching a movie adaptation of his own past, giving himself top billing surrounded by an adoring supporting cast. But I could understand why he was choosing to delude himself. The loss of status – real or perceived – is a kind of annihilation. When our children no longer need us, when work seems to have sidelined us, we fear that we will disappear. In the very places where we thought we were most visible, at our strongest, we are now disregarded.

People react to this in different ways. For some it leads to full-blown depression. For others, to anger and frustration. Like the boxer Terry Malloy in *On the Waterfront*, we cry out, 'You don't understand. I coulda had class. I coulda been a contender. I coulda been somebody.'

Feelings of low self-esteem can cause people to lash out. If we feel invisible, we will be tempted to do something – *anything* – to be noticed. Some search ever more frantically for the things they think will turn them back into a high-status individual: money, possessions, power. Others, tragically, wreck their marriages and families in order to satisfy their craving for attention.

Anything to make it feel like someone can see us again.

God #5: Rumpo, god of sex

Sub-deities: Bikini, god of lads' mags; Fnaar-fnaar, god of innuendo; Ralgex, god of bad backs.

The followers of Rumpo seem mostly to be stricken with madness. Unlike the other gods, Rumpo is rarely talked about in polite circles, or, at least, not talked about seriously. She is the subject of jokes and inference; she is constantly present, in a way, but rarely acknowledged. She does not have temples like the other gods, but in their place she has many roadside shrines, known as advertising hoardings. Many of her priests and priestesses work in modelling, but have ambitions of making it in the movies.

Apparently, there's this new type of man. He's the 'Sporno' – a man who bases his look on the ultra-ripped bodies of sportsmen and porn stars. His hair is full of product, his breakfast bowl crammed with whey protein;

he is a waxed, exfoliated and worked-out missile with one target: the ladies.

I doubt that many of my middle-aged readers will aspire to this. Our idea of protein is a pork pie.* But it says something about the godlike status of sex in our society that men should think porn stars offer something to aspire to.

Sex is everywhere. We are bombarded with sexualised images through advertising, TV, the internet, films, newspapers. But it's not just presented as a pleasure, or even a goal. It's presented as a panacea. Hollywood movies, TV shows and magazines give the impression that if the sex is great then that's all that matters. In fact, sex *is* the relationship. Sex is presented as the primary source of contact, feeling and pleasure. Anything else is just foreplay.

It is very difficult to talk honestly and openly about sex. Surveys which measure how often we have sex tend to be skewed because people tend to exaggerate so as not to appear 'indequate'. You might be interested to know that, on average, the population apparently has sex 1.55 times a week. I don't know what happens during the 0.55 bit. Maybe both partners start off, but one falls asleep.

Sex has to change in middle age. For one thing, it gets harder and harder to squeeze into that frogman's outfit. But enough of my personal issues.

There can be other problems too.

For some men, one of the most puzzling and disturbing aspects of mid-life is a loss of libido. There are many

---

* Pork, let it be noted, is a rich source of leucine, a protein which makes up one third of muscle protein and helps to stimulate repair after exercise. Eggs are also a good source of leucine. So a pork pie with an egg in it is even better.

reasons for this – the most common ones being stress and tiredness. Testosterone levels do fall as men get older, although to be honest, most of us are starting from such a ridiculously libidinous position in the first place that it probably doesn't affect things too much.

For others, the problem lies at the opposite end of the spectrum: with lust and pornography. The advent of the internet has made pornography available at the touch of a button. I'm not sure of the latest figures – and, frankly, I have no intention of trying to google any more information – but in 2010 it was reported that 12 per cent of all internet sites were pornographic and that the entire worldwide industry is worth some $4.9 billion dollars. It's hard to avoid after all: 34 per cent of internet users have experienced unwanted exposure to pornographic images through misdirected emails or unwanted 'pop ups'.[26] To coin a phrase.

But if there are problems in a relationship, if there are issues which a couple need to sort out, then their sex life is one of the first places which will feel the impact. And it is hard for men to take a balanced and relaxed view on this because they have been conditioned for so long to worship at the shrine of Eros. No man thinks that he's either bad in bed or a bad driver. (And whatever you do, don't get the two activities confused.)

Sex, of course, should be the most intimate expression of love and companionship. That's where it really works. Sex is the medium not the message. Intimacy is what we really crave. Intimacy is what will fill that yearning at our very heart.

In fact, we crave intimacy so much we are willing to pay a lot of money for people to fake it. A 2002 report estimated that British men spend an estimated £770 million per year on prostitutes, while a 2008 *Observer* survey claimed that 18 per cent of British males had visited a prostitute.*

Anyway, sex: it's not a god.

Can't think of much more to say. I said to The Wife that this was the briefest section of the book.

'Sounds appropriate,' she replied.

God #6: Prudence, god of security

Sub-deities: Stasis, god of reassurance; Ukip, god of nationalism; Retro, god of nostalgia.

The worshippers of Prudence are an anxious group of people. They spend a lot of time worrying about the future and praying to their god to protect them. They talk a lot about tradition, about the old ways of doing things, and take joy in reminiscing. They put a traditional telephone ring on their smartphone – those who have a smartphone. Some worshippers believe that their faith applies only for their own nationality or race. Doctrinal statements often begin with the line, 'I'm not racist, but . . .' Their temples are tea shops, traditional pubs and anywhere owned by the National Trust.

My friend Steve is a pretty canny guy. He's a management consultant who travels the world helping organisations to

---

* The *Observer* newspaper, I mean. There wasn't someone watching at the time.

embrace change. He is a gifted speaker and preacher. And yet he has a surprising fear.

'I find myself increasingly anxious about what might happen,' he said to me. 'I want to be prepared.'

'Prepared for what?' I asked.

'Well, what if I'm in a survival situation? I need to know that I have the right equipment on me.' Steve explained how he had done all the research. He knew how to combat hypothermia. He was researching flints and lighters so that he would always be able to make fire. He had refined his Every Day Carry – as it's called on the internet – so that he had all the equipment he needed. For his birthday, Steve asked his wife to buy him a special belt.

'It's woven out of 80 metres of paracord,' he told me. 'And it contains fishhooks and a knife.'

'Steve,' I said, 'you live in Birmingham. Are you really going to get shipwrecked somewhere on the M42?'

'You never know. The foundations of our society are so weak.'

I suppose he has a point. We are more vulnerable than we appear. And I have to admit – as a man – that his paracord belt was really cool.* But how secure against the future can we ever really be? Sometimes it just takes one event to shatter our world. This can be a big event – a bereavement, an illness, redundancy. Or it can be something as small as a missing passport. It doesn't matter.

---

* And I like being prepared. In fact, I am a man who generally carries a torch, Swiss Army knife, sewing kit, string, some duct tape wrapped around an old credit card, and a pen which also serves as a screwdriver, ruler, spirit level and stylus. Sometimes these have actually been useful.

What happens is that we suddenly realise that, no matter how much paracord we carry, we have very little control.

As I write, the UK is on a 'severe' terror alert. This alert level has been upgraded from 'substantial'. If it goes higher it reaches first 'critical' and finally 'change your trousers immediately'.

Be afraid. Be very afraid.

The activity of the first half of life is all about security. We secure ourselves against the world's ups and downs by acquiring a house, a family, a job, status, possessions, healthcare. Yet, having done that, the loudest messages from the media are messages of fear and terror. Like a conveyor belt at a sushi bar, the same threats come round and round: terrorists, immigrants, disease, global warming, crime, old age – it's the all-you-can-eat buffet of terror.

So we get this strange feeling of dissonance. We sought to protect ourselves, yet the threats seem worse than ever. We've tried to create security and stability, yet everything keeps changing. Every day brings a new technological challenge. Life has become too frantic, too fast. We are breathless from the struggle to keep up with the pace of change. I think this is one reason why 'retro' items are so popular at the moment. It's because we want to return to a golden age where the world wasn't changing every minute, and You Knew Where You Were.

The term 'nostalgia' comes from two Greek words: *nostos*, meaning 'homecoming', and *algos*, which means 'pain' or 'ache'. A painful longing for home. It was actually coined by a seventeenth-century medical student to describe anxiety symptoms displayed by Swiss mercenaries fighting away from home. Its original meaning is much more akin to homesickness. We are homesick for a lost world, a world where we once felt secure.

Sometimes a shed contains that safe world. Aberystwyth housewife Brenda Rowlands always wondered what her husband Dewi was doing in the shed. She did ask, occasionally, but he always replied, 'Just leave it,' and refused to tell her. 'I never questioned him again,' she said. When he died, aged 77, she finally went inside, to find that Dewi had been playing with his toys. Specifically, a wonderful collection of pre-World War II clockwork trains and helicopters, lead soldiers, a wooden farm and zoo animals.[27] It was his childhood, sealed in a shed-shaped container.

Of course, a great many things were better in the past. The music was better. Traffic was less. You could actually afford a house. But on the other hand, the food was rubbish, there was no internet and everyone had rickets.*

Nostalgia is one refuge. Fanaticism is another. Faced with too much change, with threatening new situations, people rush to the refuge of certainty. Fear fuels fanaticism. The belief that something we love and cherish is being eroded is one reason why so many people become more conservative as they get older. As Adam Philips wrote, 'Life becomes progressively stranger as we get older – and we become increasingly frantic to keep it familiar, to keep it in order.'[28]

---

* My grandmother used to talk fondly about the community spirit during the Blitz, which I felt rather neglected the fact that the Germans were bombing everyone at the time.

God #7: Credo, god of certainty

Sub-deities: Dogma, god of orthodox belief; Pewfilla, god of regular attendance.

The interesting thing about Credo is that he is a master of disguise. Often, his most ardent followers have no idea they are worshipping him: they believe they are worshipping another god entirely. And yet they give him money and attention and expect the rewards he promises. His temples are obvious in one way: they all look like churches. But you can only work out whether the building is dedicated to Credo or to the actual God by spending time in it. This can cause confusion for worshippers and priests alike, when they find out that even being in church is no guarantee that you're focusing on the right god.

Number seven. An appropriately sabbatarian number for this one.

Jung believed that religion has a crucial role in helping us find purpose in the second half of life. 'All great religions,' he wrote, 'hold out the promise of a life beyond . . . which makes it possible for mortal man to live the second half of life with as much purpose and aim as the first.'[29]

However, he also had painful, first-hand experience of how religion can have precisely the opposite effect. His father was a Protestant pastor who could not – or would not – bring himself to deal with the doubts and questions that seemed to undermine his faith. Unable to wrestle with God, 'he had to quarrel with somebody, so he did it with his family and himself'. Jung believed that his father was trapped in his doubts and anxieties: 'He was lonely and had no friend to talk with. At least I knew no one among our acquaintances whom I would have trusted to say the saving word. Once I heard him praying. He struggled desperately to keep his faith.'[30] What a tragic description. But how many Christians – church leaders or otherwise – have the same struggle? And how badly they, too, need a friend who will bring them the saving word.

Sadly, in my experience, a lot of men in middle age have arrived at a state of profound disillusionment with their church. And some of them are the people in charge of the place. Like my friend Steve, a church leader who increasingly found himself at odds not only with the people he was leading, but also with some of his colleagues.

'You're doing a journey that other people aren't doing,' said Steve. 'Other people want certainty, when you're starting to open up to mystery and paradox. People are saying, "Please make sure you exclude those bad people," and you're so aware of the bad part of yourself, which means you can't exclude others.'

For ministers, who work six days a week and whose evenings are filled with issues and pastoral problems, the attrition rate is very high.

'You get all these burnt-out ministers,' says Steve, 'and they're just worn out by expectations and being choked, not having the space to nurture their own souls and deal with these deeper, really important questions. When you're young, you have the energy to keep going and just ignore the doubts, but now we don't have so much energy and we can't escape those questions, and we do have to think about them and we do have to face them. We can't hide from them so easily.'

What was going on for Steve was doubt – not about his

God, but about the way God was being encountered in his church. Steve found himself in the unenviable position of exhausting himself, leading a church in a direction he didn't want to go.

'It feels horrible, as a church leader. It feels horrible that you can't be honest. Because this is a stage when you're feeling very vulnerable and very tender and you can't ... you know people want absolute certainty and they want that same old stuff, but actually that is no longer working for you any more. Your spirituality that was so great and could handle a Sunday School faith when you were a young man just doesn't work in your forties. It doesn't work.'

Steve has since worked with a lot of Christians, helping them to develop the kind of practices which can turn these dark nights into transformative experiences.

'My experience is that church becomes a worse and worse place. At first you just love it. You like worship, you like small groups, you like sermons, you like everything. But after a while, you realise that stuff doesn't really transform your character. You're receiving a lot of information, but not transformation. And it is the lack of transformation that becomes so dissatisfying at this stage of life. You start to stagnate if you're not transformed. And when you stagnate, you think, "I don't know why I'm doing this," and faith all becomes a bit of a disappointment. God becomes a disappointment, church becomes a disappointment. You're pushing everything out, because fundamentally you're disappointed with yourself.'

The worship of religious communities or institutions can be just as wrongly directed as that of any other organisation. We do not have to look very far to see churches where money has become the real god. Or churches where status is paramount, either in the form of religious titles, or in some kind of worthiness points, based on religious achievement. There are certainly churches where attendance is valued more than real participation. It's all about the numbers: as long as we have the bums on pews, the rest doesn't matter. Or churches where the real object of worship is the building or the church service itself.

Some churches worship security disguised as orthodoxy. Recently, I was due to speak at a university Christian Union meeting, but first they wanted me to sign a 'statement of faith', which I declined to do. It was nothing to do with the contents; it was the *fear* I objected to, the fear that I might say things which caused people to doubt. (Which, to be fair, I probably would, actually. But this was at a university, for heaven's sake! Isn't the purpose of university to help people use their brains?)

Those without doubts are not the faithful, but the fanatics. Actually, scratch that. Those who *appear* to be without doubt are the fanatics. They are the ones who have buried the doubt deep, who have suppressed it, hidden it beneath ever-thicker layers of orthodox activity and statements. In one of my favourite films, *Tinker, Tailor, Soldier, Spy*, the hero George Smiley recalls an attempt to get the Russian spy commander Karla to defect during the time of the Stalinist purges. Despite being betrayed by his own leaders, despite knowing he would most likely be killed, Karla refuses to defect. And from this, Smiley discerns his fatal flaw: fanaticism.

'That's how I know he can be beaten,' says Smiley.

'Because he's a fanatic. And the fanatic is always conceal-ing a secret doubt.' John le Carré, who wrote the novel on which the film is based, once described Smiley as 'a committed doubter'.[31]

'Wherever belief reigns, doubt lurks in the background,' wrote Jung. 'But thinking people welcome doubt, it serves them as a valuable stepping stone to better knowledge.'[32] Jesus always reserved his sternest words for those who were certain of their own orthodoxy and righteousness. Whereas for those people who admitted their failings and their fears – for the committed doubters – he had nothing but compassion and love.

He told a story of two men praying at the temple. One was a Pharisee, a member of the grass-roots holiness movement in Judaism at the time. The other was a tax collector, who would have been viewed as a collaborator with the occupying forces. The Pharisee congratulated himself that he was 'not like other people: thieves, rogues, adulterers, or even like this tax collector. I fast twice a week; I give a tenth of all my income.' The tax collector, standing alone and hoping not to be noticed, 'would not even look up to heaven', but instead beat his breast and murmured, 'God, be merciful to me, a sinner!' In the end, said Jesus, it is the tax collector who is OK with God, 'for all who exalt themselves will be humbled, but all who humble themselves will be exalted' (Luke 18:9–14).

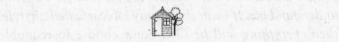

All the wrong dreams

Many men feel like failures in their middle age, not because they are failures in themselves, but because their gods have failed them. Perhaps you do not see your own personal gods mentioned here. I am sure there are any number of ready-to-worship false gods out there. But all false gods have two things in common. First, they will all let you down, and second, *the gods do not care*.

'The mass of men,' wrote Thoreau, 'live lives of quiet desperation.' It is a disturbing thing, that dark night moment when you realise that the gods to whom you have given your life have let you down. And the reason that it occurs in middle age more than at any other time is, I think, because in the first half of life we can still hold out the hope that they will deliver on their promises. There is still plenty of time for our worship to be rewarded. But by middle age, as we've seen, our illusions have gone. We have seen the best that these gods can do, and found it wanting.

When men become aware of the failure of their gods, they react in different ways. Some go into denial. *There's nothing wrong. It's all OK. I'll just retreat to my shed.* Some recognise that something has gone wrong, but project that failure onto others. *It's her fault, she doesn't understand me. If I can change my job/car/wife/hairstyle, then everything will be OK.* Some choose to redouble their efforts. *Worship harder! It can't be the god's fault, it must be me.* And so they work harder, earn more, believe with an ever greater, ever more gritted-teeth certainty.

I don't believe that any of these approaches really work, because beneath the surface the fires are raging. All that fear, frustration and anger must come out somewhere. The last time I went to a football match was a mid-week game. Just before kick-off a man came in and sat next to me. He was still in his suit: evidently he had come straight from work. And from the moment the team emerged from the tunnel, he never stopped shouting, the veins on his temples throbbing with rage. I have never seen a man so angry. Everything was wrong: the team, the referee, the tactics . . . But I couldn't help thinking that the real cause of his anger lay elsewhere, in his life outside the football stadium. The team was merely the outlet for his rage.

I think that much of the grumpiness of mid-life springs from this kind of mis-directed frustration. Believe me, I can get angry about a lot of things – including but not limited to the M25, plastic shrink-wrap packaging, celebrity authors, internet advertising, the idea that radio phone-in programmes should be taken seriously, the England cricket team/football team/rugby team, etc., etc. But this anger does not really stem from the things themselves, but from my own frustration. I often end up taking out my anger on some inanimate object – shouting at the computer or banging the steering wheel of the car – not because that will solve anything, but because there is such a lot of anger inside me, and it *must* come out.

The wrong gods will always fail us. For some men this leads to anger and frustration. For others it is expressed in fear and anxiety. We lie awake at night worrying about money, about where the next job is coming from, about what will happen to us in the future. We feel helpless, isolated, trapped. The German term for 'mid-life crisis' is *Torschlusspanik*, literally 'door-shut-panic', fear of being on the wrong side of a closing gate. 'It's too late,' we think. 'The train has left the station, the horse has bolted. I've been left behind.'

Sometimes we just feel unhappy. Very, very unhappy. We cry during films – which would be OK, but it's during the credits. We put on Mozart's *Requiem* to cheer ourselves up. Sometimes this manifests itself as depression, but more often I've met men who just seem to be unhappy at life in general. They don't express it in those terms, they normally have something else they've been let down by – church, work, children. But the unhappiness and failure is deep inside them.

One problem is that we have been misinformed by Thomas Jefferson. Well, him and the rest of the American founding fathers. Not only did they make the signal error of seeking to be free from Glorious British Rule™, but they put in 'the pursuit of happiness' as one of the three fundamental rights, the other two being life and Coca-Cola. Sorry, liberty. But what on earth does that mean? How do you 'pursue happiness'? I remember my father saying to me, right after he had walked out on my mother, 'I have a right to be happy.' Even as a fairly self-obsessed 18-year-old, I could see that there were problems with this. Because in that case, at least, happiness was a zero-sum game. His 'happiness' was achieved only at the cost of someone else's misery.

I'm not knocking happiness. I enjoy being happy.

Although, as a middle-aged man, paradoxically, some-times I am at my most happy when I am extremely grumpy. But the goal of life is not happiness. That's a by-product. When Jesus listed the kind of people who should be happy, he included those who mourn, the poor, the humble, those who are desperate for justice and those who are persecuted for following him. They are happy not because they have pursued personal pleasure, but because they have given their lives for a greater goal. All those people, in Jesus' view, were happy because they did not put happiness first.

Which brings us back to the scribe who asked Jesus that question about the most important commandment. When he heard Jesus' answer to his question, he agreed – loving God and loving your neighbour as yourself was more important, he affirmed, than 'all whole burnt-offer-ings and sacrifices'. Which, considering that the scribe's job pretty much revolved around the sacrificial system and the temple, was a big statement.

And in response, Jesus told him something very surprising: 'You are not far from the kingdom of God' (Mark 12:33-34).

The negative feelings that we have in middle age are a great and powerful truth. As Gerard Hughes says, 'The facts are kind and God is in the facts.'[33] These feelings alert us that something is wrong. It is good to realise that the objects of our worship are not going to deliver on their promises, and that our achievements, however good they are, will not deliver the deep satisfying life that we crave. Because once you have identified all the gods who have failed, you can start to look for one who might succeed.

The mid-life crisis, if you want to call it that, is a call. That is what the word means, actually. The word 'crisis' derives from the Greek word *krinein*, 'to make a decision'. When we undergo this dark night, we have a choice to make. We can keep our sadness, anger, feelings of frustration and failure and loss. We can choose to deny that anything is wrong. We can blame the whole thing on other people and find someone new, with whom we can start again.

Or we can try something completely different.

Arthur Miller, in his shed, wrote the play *Death of a Salesman*. It tells the tragic story of a salesman, Willy Loman, who desperately tries to keep up the appearance of success when his whole world is falling apart around him. For years he has been putting on the persona of a successful, popular, go-getting salesman, but events start to shatter his lies. First he suffers a pay cut and is forced to work solely on commission, then he is fired. His sons fail to live up to the impossible dreams he projected onto them. Finally, tragically, he takes his own life. At his funeral, his son Biff cries out, 'He had the wrong dreams . . . He never knew who he was.'

We have all the wrong dreams. We feel like we have lost, but the truth is that we were playing a game we could never win. What we need is a new purpose, a new set of dreams, a God who will not fail. And it is towards him that I want to turn next.

But we will need a different approach. 'We cannot live the afternoon of life according to the programme of life's morning,' wrote Jung. 'For what was great in the morning will be little at evening, and what in the morning was true will at evening have become a lie.'[34] Or, as Richard Rohr puts it, 'You cannot walk the second journey with first journey tools. You need a whole new toolkit.'[35]

And as a middle-aged man, I *love* the idea of getting a whole new toolkit.

PART TWO

THE RESPONSE

*The world breaks everyone and afterward
many are strong at the broken places.*

Ernest Hemingway, *A Farewell to Arms*

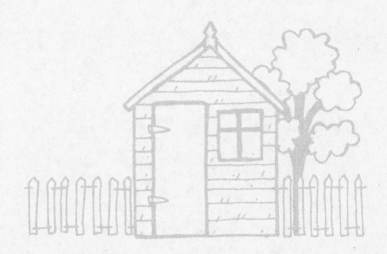

PART THREE

THE RESPONSE

The world breaks everyone and afterward
many are strong at the broken places.

Ernest Hemingway, *A Farewell to Arms*

He had watched the procession all day from the top of the ridge. Men and women, goats, donkeys and camels laden with goods, all of them fording the river and heading west. And now, as the sun was setting, there was just the one man down there, waiting alone. Looking lost.

He shrugged. One of old Abram's children, apparently. Odd lot. Never could make sense of those people. He checked his own few goats and lay down to sleep.

Something woke him in the middle of the night. A noise. Thunder, perhaps. But when he looked around there were no rainclouds to be seen. Instead the moon was bright and big as a platter, and he could see clearly down to the river. With a start he realised the man was still there. But no longer alone. He was standing with his arms clasped around another figure. A big man. Ankle deep in the water, the two of them rocked back and forth, moving slowly, straining against – or towards – one another.

And as he looked, he realised that he could not tell whether they were wrestling, embracing, or dancing.

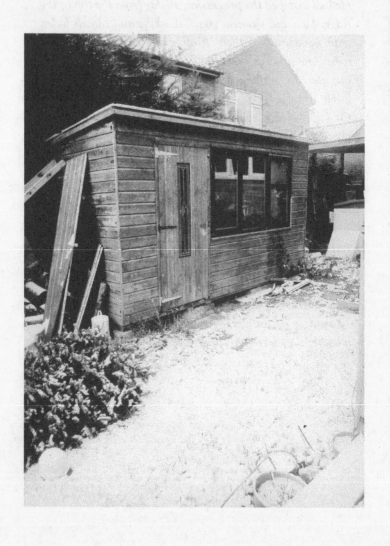

5

WRESTLING

The call to adventure

Rebuilding the shed was both exciting and ridiculously hard work.

Fortunately the floor was strong and sound. That was the strongest part of the building. It was sound and dry and it gave me confidence that at least the foundations were solid. Before working on the windows, I insulated the floor and put new boards down. At least there was something to build on.

The walls, though, were a different matter. Nothing in this building was square. Nothing was on a right angle. Over the years the shed had slumped and sagged and leaned in one way or the other, so cutting wood to fit these various angles was a challenge. If you start off-square, then everything is wrong. But, as they tend to say in middle management, 'we are where we are'. And I was in a shabby, run-down wooden shack. In the snow.

Yes, *snow*. The day after the first windows went in, I put another window in the end wall of the shed and rebuilt the door. And it snowed all the time. I became a writer in order to avoid outdoor work, heavy lifting, the cold. Now, here I was, standing in the freezing snow. In retrospect, starting the work at the end of autumn was not the cleverest move. I found myself working in the dark and the cold. No matter how many layers I put on, I was still freezing. By this stage I had on a thermal vest, a sweatshirt, a woollen lumberjack shirt and a jacket. On my head was one of those Russian tank commander style hats. I looked like a kind of Soviet Michelin man. Even before I started cutting great holes in it, the shed offered no protection from the elements.

But I comforted myself with the fact that I was not just rebuilding a shed. I was responding to a call. And that needed courage.

A couple of years ago, a little while after my minor falling apart, I went to lead a writers' retreat at a centre in Yorkshire, where I spent some time with an old friend of mine. He gave me two words which he thought I needed and which, indeed, every writer needs: 'honesty' and 'courage'. Those have become my mantra, my watchwords over the succeeding years: honesty, and courage.

Last Christmas, one of my daughters gave me a carpenter's pencil, a long, blue, flattened tube. Now I see that, even in her permanently plugged-in adolescent state, this child had somehow discerned the journey on which I would have to embark. The child is clearly a visionary. Shame I can't remember which one it was who gave me the present. Anyway, she knew the journey would require much sawing and nailing and hammering and marking things on bits of wood. 'Travail' and 'travel' have the same word as their root. All journeys are meant to be hard work.

The squashed shape of a carpenter's pencil is, apparently, designed to stop it rolling away down a roof. Its width makes it stronger and less likely to break in a toolbox. The width of the graphite allows you to draw

either thick or thin lines depending on how you hold it.*
You can't sharpen a carpenter's pencil with a normal
sharpener, you need to use a knife. It is, of all pencils, the
most manly.

Once all the windows were in, it was time to start
adding insulation and putting up interior walls. When the
first panel was in place I took my manly carpenter's pencil
and wrote two words on it: 'honesty' and 'courage'.

Into the depths

The call to adventure always comes as a surprise.

Many of our myths reflect this. In *Aladdin*, the hero is
living from hand to mouth on the street when he is offered
the opportunity to descend into the cave and retrieve a
treasure. In Bunyan's *Pilgrim's Progress*, the hero,
Christian, has his life disrupted by a vision of his home
city being destroyed by fire. In the *Aeneid*, Aeneas is
standing among the ruins of Troy when he sees a vision of
his lost wife, Creusa,† who tells him that he must find a
new home, in a land far to the West, across 'a great waste
of ocean'.

---

* There's a Wikipedia entry on it. Gripping reading. Actually, the
oldest pencil in existence is a carpenter's pencil, found in the attic of
a seventeenth-century house in Germany. See http://www.pencilpages.
com/gallery/oldest.htm.
† She later went on to develop a range of cookware.

Jacob's grandfather received a call as well. I don't know what life was like for Abram at the time. He was settled in Haran when one day God spoke to him: 'Go from your country and your kindred and your father's house to the land that I will show you' (Genesis 12:1). God has a new purpose for him; Abram responds to the call.*

My favourite example of this is in the magnificent *LEGO Movie*. The hero, Emmet, thinks that his life is fine. 'Everything is Awesome', as the corporate mantra goes. There are hints of uncertainty: on the early morning TV programme, he hears the villain of the piece say, 'Obey the rules. Or you'll be put to sleep.' For a moment this disturbs him, but he is distracted by the latest episode of a TV programme called *Where Are My Pants?* Emmet lives his life according to the instructions. But then he has a cataclysmic event. He falls down a hole, finds the Piece of Resistance, accidentally becomes the Chosen One and his adventure begins. But before that his life was proceeding serenely and untroubled. Everything was awesome.

The word 'catastrophe' is a Greek word which literally means 'a down stroke'. And we are called to go down into the depths, into the cave, to see what treasures there are waiting. Because, in the words of Jung, 'The treasure which the hero fetches from the dark cavern is *life*: it is himself.'[36]

The call to new life involves a descent. Certainly that was true for Jacob. The geographical details of the story show that Jacob took his wives, children and livestock

---

* Abram was 75 when God called him. Since he lived, according to the Bible, to the age of 175, he was in early middle age at this point.

across the Jabbok, a river in eastern Canaan which enters the Jordan about 23 miles north of the Dead Sea. The Jabbok starts at 1,900 feet above sea level and descends, through deep canyons and ravines, to 115 feet below sea level. Jacob is literally in the depths.

He is 'low' in every way. He cannot sleep. He is not thinking clearly. The story is full of confused movement. Fording a river is risky in the daylight; at night it's just desperate. He seems to cross with them and then return. He sends them on, but stays behind. What is going through his mind? Is he, perhaps, tempted to slip away, to melt into the hills and never come back?

At this point, the lowest point in his life, Jacob has a decision to make. Jacob had been running for most of his life, but in the Jabbok river that night he decided to stand and fight. The biblical story is full of puns. The river is the *yabbok*; the word for 'wrestle' is *yeabeq*. It's related to the Hebrew word for 'dust' – *abeq*.[37] Jacob is prepared to get his hands dirty.

We cannot move into the second half of life unless we are prepared to stand and fight. Too many men, I think, prefer 'flight' to 'fight': they avoid the conflict entirely in the hope that things will sort themselves out, or, worse, they run away and make the same mistakes all over again.

On my way home the other day I saw an old acquaintance. Steve – as I shall call him – used to be in our church, until he left his wife for a much younger woman. We're roughly the same age, I think, but what made me take notice was that he was walking along pushing a push-chair, with a baby in it. And he looked so miserable. I wondered what was going through his head. Was this really what he wanted? Was this the freedom he yearned for? Because to me he just looked like someone who was making the same mistakes all over again.

Looks, of course, can be deceiving. You can have a new baby at any point in your life. I am sure that child will be loved, but, for me, Steve looked very much like someone who chose flight over fight.

'One who runs away from his encounter with spiritual reality cannot be transformed,' writes John Sanford.[38] The first thing we have to do is to follow Jacob's example and have a good wrestle. Paradoxically, we will never find real peace unless we accept God's invitation to fight.

That fight will be revealing. It will show us the truth about ourselves, and that can be painful and scary. We have worn our masks for so long that taking them off is like stripping away layers of skin. It takes honesty to see ourselves as we really are and it takes courage to identify what we are really afraid of.

And the fight will show us that we cannot win in our own strength. Jacob was a strong man, but when it came to the final round he was beaten easily. But that's OK. We have to be defeated by God, because it is only in that defeat that we will find victory.

Honesty and courage. 'The facts are kind and God is in the facts.'

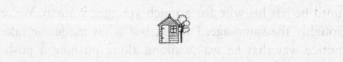

Flotsam and jetsam

Gradually the shed began to take shape.

I constructed the interior walls out of whatever I could find: bits of old laminate flooring, old packing cases rescued from skips, builders' plywood, cut-up bits of old furniture. I panelled the wall above one window with the front of an old drawer that used to be in the girls' room when they were small. It's bright yellow and blue and still has kitten and butterfly stickers on it and a label saying 'horses'.

I rebuilt the door and lined it and put into it a piece of stained glass from our old front door. Over the door I embedded the '1000' badge from my old Morris Traveller. As the shed became more secure, I started to put furniture back in. At one end, to serve as a tool cupboard, I put the bottom half of an old dresser which I put together when The Wife and I were first married. On some days it was actually warm enough (well, with the help of a fan heater) to sit and write. For a temporary work table I used a folding picnic table which I have kept since I was young. I used to sit with my brother at this table when we went caravanning with our parents. We would spend hours together, making up Airfix kits and painting model soldiers. The table still has the traces of old Humbrol paints on it, small flecks of green and red. It's forty years old, this table, and still functioning perfectly. Although the underside is a little dusty, and some of the laminate is falling off. Maybe I shouldn't push this metaphor too far . . .

One way or another, there was a lot of my past in this building, a lot of the flotsam and jetsam from my life. The past is always with us. But who am I *now*? That is the question. And who am I going to be?

The two questions

God places before us two questions: 'Who are you?' and 'What are you afraid of?'

At one point in the fight, Jacob appears to have the upper hand. His opponent even asks Jacob to release him! Jacob, spotting an opening, immediately demands his prize: a blessing. No surprise there – that's what he's been conditioned to seek out. What was Jacob looking for now: more land, more sons, more livestock? The stranger doesn't answer, anyway. Instead, he asks Jacob a question: 'What is your name?'

It's a strange question, when you come to think about it. This, after all, is God. He's already met Jacob several times before in dreams. He's not here by accident, we assume; he didn't just stumble across Jacob in that river. No, he chose to come and wrestle with Jacob. He knows *exactly* who he is fighting.

But names in the Bible are not just labels: they are expressions of character and purpose. Jacob's name – 'supplanter', 'grasper' – was also his nature. Of course God knows Jacob's true identity. What he's interested in is whether Jacob knows it. What God is asking Jacob is,

'Who do you think you are? What are you like?' He's asking Jacob to confess his true nature.

God knows all about us, but he's really interested to find out what we have discovered about ourselves. I have learnt a lot from a friend and teacher called Trevor Hudson. One phrase of his which has really stuck with me is, 'God is always interested in what you haven't told him yet.' The famous sign in the forecourt of the Temple of Apollo at Delphi said, 'Know yourself.' We spend a lot of our lives in what Trevor calls 'impression-management'. What a potent phrase. All that time and energy trying to manage other people's impressions of us. We want to be seen as clever, competent, important, self-controlled. We don't want them to see the real us. And they're doing the same. Everyone plays the game.

Of course, to a certain extent we have to do this. People want professionalism. As a freelancer, I have to manage the impressions of my clients. I can't go into a meeting visibly crippled with self-doubt, dressed in my dressing gown and slippers and clutching a flask of whisky. It would not make the right impression, although some days it might be a more honest reflection of my internal state. Some of our persona is necessary. If I went into a solicitor's office to find that he was wearing a red false nose, huge shoes and a wig, I might think that there was something odd about him. We don't want to find our doctor unshaven, smelly and sitting there in his underpants. Or, indeed, anyone else's underpants.

The persona serves a necessary social function. But the problem with the persona is that it is not us. In offering a presentable face to the world, we have to suppress the bits of us which we think the world does not want to see. Behind the mask, all kinds of terrors and anxieties and glories and wonders may be lurking. There is another, deeper us, the one who is only revealed in the dark night moments. This is one of the reasons why so many middle-aged men feel split in two: there is a vast difference between the person we present to the world and the one who lies awake at night.

Our lives, like Jacob's, are characterised by duplicity. Sometimes our assumed persona masks actual lies and self-delusion or, at least, a lack of self-knowledge. Sometimes the persona we show to the world is just the idea that everything is 'OK'. We look fine and behave normally, but we are really scared and sad and really, really tired, because duplicity is so exhausting. As any *Star Trek* fan will tell you, it drains a lot of energy when you have the deflector shields set to full.

The only way that this will change is if we can come to a point where we do not have to pretend, where we do not mind the world seeing the real us, because the real us is nothing to be ashamed of. So, how do we do this?

First, like Jacob, we need to find a space where we can be alone to wrestle. Just us and God. No distractions. No appointments to go to. Some people choose to go on a long walk. Some will go on retreat. Churches are good places to sit and think, giving us, in Francis Spufford's words, 'the hush in which we can bear to find out what we're like'.[39] The *really* holy ones get to sit in a shed.

But wherever it is, we need to find a place where we can answer God's question, 'Who are you?' This is a life and death question, in the sense that it is the first step on moving from death to abundant life. In the Gospels, Jesus encounters a man who is literally living among the dead. Mark describes him as being uncontrollable: no one could secure him, not even with chains. He has turned a terrible, self-harming fury and despair on himself. This is a man who is tearing himself apart. Jesus casts the demons out of him, but he does so with a single, really important question: 'What is your name?' (Mark 5:9)

It is the 'powers' within the man who answer. But perhaps the question was simpler than that. It's the same question, really, that God asked Jacob a couple of thousand years earlier. 'What are you called?' *Who are you?*

Perhaps you know what it is to live among the tombs, to be exiled to a place of dead dreams and hopes. Perhaps you, like this poor man, howl and rage in despair. Maybe you feel like you have a legion of different personas, a man of a thousand faces, all facing in different directions so that you feel torn apart by the warfare within.

Who are you? What is your nature? If God asked you the same question, what would you say? Jacob owned up to what he had become. Esau always thought 'Jacob' – 'supplanter' – was the perfect name for him (Genesis 27:36), and in this moment Jacob agrees with his brother. He is a liar, a cheat, always grasping for the blessing.

And having admitted that, much to his surprise, he finds out that wasn't the real answer at all.

Who are you?

Who are we? Well, for starters, we are not our jobs.

Go to any party or get into any conversation with a stranger, and it is not long before one man will ask another, 'What do you do?'

Now, the correct answer to this question is another question: 'What do I do, when?' I mean, I do many things. Sometimes I sleep, sometimes I eat. I scratch myself, drink coffee, lie on the sofa watching the rugby, work on my shed, pray, worry where the next job is coming from, drink more coffee . . .

But we don't mean that. We mean, 'What do you do for a living?' To which you reply, 'I am a doctor', 'I am a software engineer', 'I am a teacher.'

You see what's happened? When asked about what we do, we reply with what our job is. We have to let go of the idea that we are what we do. It skews so many facets of our lives. For men, the 'What do you do?' question is often an attempt to place a new acquaintance on the organisation chart of life, to work out their standing in the herd. Is this someone I should be anxious about? Is this someone who could help me? Is this someone I should pay attention to? I do quite well on this one, because when I reply, airily, 'Oh, I'm a writer, actually,' it's clear that what I am actually saying is, 'Hah! In your face, corporate bloke with your BMW and your suit and your well-paid job. I am not a slave to "the man". I am a bohemian free spirit. I am a *writer*.' That's the subtext in my mind, anyway.

The 'What do you do?' question has some of its roots in our need for status, and it can lead us into those silly status-battle conversations. I met a guy the other day. I'll call him Steve, because I can't actually remember his real name anyway. Steve worked with creating sustainable communities, or something like that. It sounded really good, worthwhile work, but our entire conversation – and I use the word loosely – consisted of him asking me questions to which he already knew the answer, but I didn't. It was more like a job interview. Or the weirdest pub quiz ever. 'What do you think about the situation in Nigeria?' 'How much energy does your house use?' 'What do you think is the main problem facing society today?' And every time I ventured an opinion, he shook his head and said, 'No, I'll tell you what it is . . .' By the end of it I was making up answers. *Seven. No, forty-two. No, wait a minute, is it Bolton Wanderers?*

It was exhausting and I couldn't help wondering, at the end of it, why Sustainable Steve needed to talk in this way. What was lacking in his life that meant he had to 'win' this conversation? Worse, every unanswerable question was about his job. When I tried to ask him about himself, he wasn't interested. And he was only interested in me insofar as he could demonstrate my ignorance.

Equally, I'm sure we've all had those kinds of conversations where it becomes quite clear early on that the person talking to you has already dismissed you and really wants to get out of this chat as soon as possible. You are not going to be of use to them, so they spend the whole conversation looking over your shoulder for someone more important. We have probably all done this kind of thing as well.

We are not our jobs. Nor are we our activities. We fill our lives with busyness: meetings, appointments, conferences, business trips. I remember once being at a planning meeting for a conference and trying to get a diary date together with some church ministers. It almost became a competition about who had the busiest schedule, as if how busy we were proved something about our importance.

Such is the importance of work to our lives and our sense of who we are, that it can completely define us. But I am not my job. That is just the 'something' that I do to earn money. It's a very important something, it matters a lot to me and I really enjoy it, but it could go away and I would still be here.

We are not what we do. And we are not what we own. We've been sold this idea of 'lifestyle' as if our possessions can shape our entire existence. We buy into this – in all senses of that phrase. We have already looked at how adverts sell us emotions and feelings, but in some cases they also sell us identity. I am an Apple user, which for years enabled me to look with withering scorn on all those poor PC users. They didn't 'think different', as the Apple ads so ungrammatically put it. We bolster ourselves by deriding others. We pride ourselves on our wisdom and choices by mocking or belittling the choices of others. Consumerist economies stay afloat 'by manipulating the low self-esteem of their consumers and by creating spiritual expectations through material means'.[40] Our purchases somehow make us feel better about ourselves. But as Francis Spufford writes, 'Your life is not a product; you cannot expect to unwrap it, and place it in an advantageous corner of your Docklands flat, and admire the way the halogen spots on your lighting track gleam on its sleek sides.'[41]

Jesus himself warned against identifying what we own with who we are: 'Take care! Be on your guard against all kinds of greed; for one's life does not consist in the abundance of possessions' (Luke 12:15).

You are not what you own. Jacob had to let go of all he owned before he could find out who he really was. No one can take their possessions with them into the dark night. You can't wrestle God with your arms full.

We are not what we look like. One of George Orwell's last notes in his notebook was, 'At 50, everyone has the face he deserves.'[42]Orwell's face certainly bore the impression of a hard life. But increasingly, we all want to cheat.

I think men are under less pressure than women when it comes to appearance, but we are susceptible to this nevertheless. Television and movies bombard us with images of handsome men, impossibly buff and with beautiful physiques. It's interesting to notice, particularly, how muscular leading men are now. When you see Clark Gable or Errol Flynn bare-chested you notice how relatively thin they were. But now, every actor works out. I'm not saying that appearance is unimportant. I sometimes meet men who say, 'I don't care what I look like,' and I think, 'Well, yes, but you don't have to look at yourself.' But we are not the expensive suit we wear, or the Grecian 2000 in our hair, or the six-pack. Nor, indeed, are we the baldness, the beer gut or the much-loved shabby shapeless cardigan.

Finally, and most importantly, we are not our failures.

Why is it that we find it so hard to remember the good times, and so easy to remember the bad times? Of course, as an Englishman, I am finely attuned to embarrassment and shame, but even adjusting for that, it's amazing how much my past failings clutter my memory. The good things – the acts of kindness, the jokes, the fun, the moments when I am actually quite nice – all those are fugitive, fleeting. Instead, what clings to my memory are the times when I did or said something wrong, those moments of acute shame and embarrassment. I am covered with the scar tissue of my failings. I carry them around with me, *The Worst Hits of Nick Page*. In 3D and full surround sound. And in the dark night it is those which replay in my head: the words I can never unsay, the deeds I can never undo.

The Bible calls these failings 'sin'. The modern world, though, doesn't really get the concept of sin. It thinks the concept antiquated. Folklore. When it talks of sin, it equates the word with 'a bit of naughtiness', like having an extra portion of ice cream or one drink too many. You know, it's bad, but it's not evil. The Bible, however, refuses to play down the problem. Sin is not mere over-indulgence. It is failure and selfishness and wrongdoing. At its core, all sin is a move in the wrong direction, a movement away from God. And whether you're the Pope, a priest, a policeman or a paedophile, we all do it.

The world doesn't understand the concept of sin, but it really grasps the concept of shame. Oh yes, we know how to shame people. We know how to plaster people's failures and mistakes and plain bad deeds all over the internet. And that means, however far they run they cannot escape the shame. The internet documents every detail of our lives. Employers increasingly check our

Facebook profile for evidence of wrongdoing or thought-crime. And once it's there, it's there for life. But the Bible says that sin is not permanent. It does not have to define us. Christianity agrees that we are all failures, but then tells us that those failures do not have to stay around for ever. No one is free from sin, but no one is beyond forgiveness and the grace and love of God. This is really the radical message at the heart of Christianity: no one is denied a new start. No one.

Jesus was always being criticised because he spent so much time with sinners. 'Haven't you read their Facebook pages?' the religious people would ask him. 'Haven't you seen the kind of pictures they've posted? Haven't you googled them and seen what they have done? It's all in the archives.' Of course he knew. He *always* knew. It just never made any difference. In the course of a taboo-busting conversation with a Samaritan woman (John 4), Jesus reveals that he knows about her past, the five husbands she's gone through and the sixth that she's working on. And *still* he gives her his attention and talks with her and jokes with her and drinks the water she gives him. So when she runs back into the village, it is the fact that he knows all about her yet still has time for her that changes everything: 'Come and see a man who told me everything I have ever done!' she shouts to the neighbours – most of whom already knew what she had done and had made their minds up about her a long time ago.

They might have made their minds up about her, but Jesus hadn't. He always sees people's potential. Jesus never gets angry or upset at sinners. He reserves that for people who do not think they are sinners at all. Indeed,

Jesus was always going round forgiving people – even when they didn't actually ask for it; even on the cross, when humanity's ability to opt for the grubbiest, most brutal path was at its zenith, even then he still offered forgiveness.

And just as we are not 'everything I have ever done', neither are we all the things that have been done to us. *We are not our wounds.* It is easy to get trapped into a permanent victimhood, especially as we get older. As injustices – real or perceived – are heaped upon us, they shape us, they become us. So we whine about our bad luck or our parents or authority or our work or . . . well, you get the point. When Jesus' disciples asked him for a template to help them pray, he included this clause: 'And forgive us our sins, for we ourselves forgive everyone indebted to us' (Luke 11:4). He spoke about it several times, in fact. In Mark's Gospel he said, 'Whenever you stand praying, forgive, if you have anything against anyone; so that your Father in heaven may also forgive you your trespasses' (Mark 11:25).

At the end of his life, Jung was asked by one of his 'disciples' what his pilgrimage had been. He said, 'My journey consisted in climbing down ten thousand ladders so that now, at the end of my life I can extend the hand of friendship to this little clod of earth that I am.'[43]

Forgiving ourselves and forgiving others: the two activities are hard to tell apart. Sometimes, indeed, the issue is precisely that the 'other' we cannot forgive is ourselves. We confess our sins and then cling onto them. We do not really believe that it is possible to get rid of them. We are harder on ourselves than God is. The letter of John talks of the habit of self-condemnation, of how 'our hearts condemn us', and assures us that 'God is greater than our hearts, and he knows everything' (1 John 3:20).

Everything we've ever done, in fact.

The shadow side

Jacob answered God's question with honesty and courage. It was through being honest about his true nature that he was able to be transformed. We are not defined by our failings, but it is really important to identify them – not so that we can use them to beat ourselves up with, but so that we can become aware of who we really are.

Jung called this stuff the 'shadow'. He saw it as the darker, instinctual part of the psyche, that part of us we suppress or deny or fail to recognise. But he also believed that there was energy locked away in the shadow. It's like anti-matter in *Star Trek*. Or positive and negative poles on a battery. Once we acknowledge the shadow part of ourselves, we become clearer about our own choices, our own behaviour. And if we are ever going to become whole people, we have to deal with this shadow side of ourselves. If we reject it, or suppress it, or, worst of all, fear to even go near it, we can never be whole. This is because we will most likely have to carry on dealing with all this crap for the rest of our lives. God does not magically erase the desires which lead to sin. We remain free, capable of making choices. Forgiveness of sin is not like some kind of spiritual amputation, where the very desire itself is magically removed. That's not how it works. It couldn't possibly work that way, because sin is what happens when good and healthy emotions get warped or misdirected. It's to do with things that are intrinsically part of us – but which are directed the wrong way. This is why Richard Rohr writes, 'I do not think you should get rid of your sin until you have learned what it has to teach you.'[44] Our sin, properly confessed and identified, has much to teach us about ourselves. It helps us understand our motivations and vulnerabilities; it helps us to understand what it is we are scared of.

In the artistic triumph that is the Arnold Schwarzenegger film *Predator,* a group of soldiers is being hunted by an invisible foe. The Predator is impossible to fight, because you can't see it. It is only when Arnie destroys its ability to turn invisible that it can be thoroughly Schwarzeneggered. And when Arnie sees it, he says, 'What the hell *are* you?' But the alien Predator just distorts his answer and throws it back: 'What the hell are *you*?' You have to give shape to the Predators in your life. And just like the eponymous Predator, as we question our darker side, it will, in turn, ask questions of us. It is important, then, to look unflinchingly at our shadow side. Some of them are our failings – our sins. But there is another class of predatory feelings which also need to be named and given shape: our fears.

I believe that we need to turn anxiety into fear. Anxiety is generalised. Anxiety is like a fog, and you can't fight a fog, but fears – fears are specific. So as well as asking yourself about your failings, ask yourself about your fears. What, exactly, are you afraid of? For me, I am learning to look at my fear more critically. And either I discover that there is something I can do about it, or I discover that there is nothing I can really do, in which case my worrying won't make any difference.

Jesus spoke more about fear than virtually anything else. He was continually telling his followers not to be worried or afraid or anxious. One of his most famous speeches about it is recorded in Matthew's Gospel:

Therefore I tell you, do not worry about your life, what you will eat or what you will drink, or about your body, what you will wear. Is not life more than food, and the body more than clothing? Look at the birds of the air; they neither sow nor reap nor gather into barns, and yet your heavenly Father feeds them. Are you not of more value than they? And can any of you by worrying add a single hour to your span of life? ... Therefore do not worry, saying, 'What will we eat?' or 'What will we drink?' or 'What will we wear?' For it is the Gentiles who strive for all these things; and indeed your heavenly Father knows that you need all these things. But strive first for the kingdom of God and his righteousness, and all these things will be given to you as well. So do not worry about tomorrow, for tomorrow will bring worries of its own. Today's trouble is enough for today. (Matthew 6:25-27, 31-34)

This is one of those bits of the Gospels where I put the initials TOKFJ in the margin: 'That's OK For Jesus'. I mean, this was a man who could do miracles, so of course he didn't worry about these sorts of things.

And yet he is right. There is very little in life that we can truly control. There are all kinds of greater powers which can affect us for better or for worse. I can try to adopt a healthy lifestyle, but ultimately I can't control whether or not I succumb to cancer or dementia or Parkinson's disease or any of the other crappy stuff that life throws at us. In Jesus' words, 'Can any of us by worrying add a single hour to life?'

Now, I don't want to be all simplistic about this. I have read a lot on this subject and meditated and prayed and done all that stuff, and yet there are still times when I get that churning in my guts, that sinking feeling when the car goes wrong again, or I don't know where the next bit of work is coming from, or when I look ahead and imagine all the worst things that could happen. All that dark night stuff. The only reliable thing I have found for dealing with these fears, apart from a bottle of Sauvignon Blanc, is to attend to the words of Jesus and realise that I matter. Later on in Matthew's Gospel, Jesus says, 'Are not two sparrows sold for a penny? Yet not one of them will fall to the ground unperceived by your Father. And even the hairs of your head are all counted. So do not be afraid; you are of more value than many sparrows' (Matthew 10:29-31).

So when God asks, 'Who are you?' our first task is to answer honestly. 'I am Nick. I am a 54-year-old man, who loves his wife and children, but who is scared a lot of the time. I try to write the best words I can, but often they aren't up to the task I set myself. I am an idiot who thinks that building a shed could solve any of his problems. I speak too often without thinking, I try to be funny without being cruel or mean, but sometimes I fail. I am prey to lust and greed and selfishness and anger. Although not necessarily in that order and rarely all at once. Is that enough to be going on with?'

Once we have 'named' ourselves, then we can allow God to rename us. When God asked Jacob who he was, Jacob offered up his own, raw, honest understanding of his nature: he was what he had always been – a supplanter, a grasper.

And God is so pleased with him that he does the most loving thing he can. He defeats him.

Skip-raiding

The Wife insisted that I could not spend much on the shed. Not when there were other things in the house that needed proper spending on and proper attention. Little things like, oh, a shower that leaked, a bedroom which hadn't been redecorated since the Bronze Age, mattresses which were marginally less comfortable than concrete.

Although I thought that this showed a rather frivolous and unspiritual view of life, I agreed, and thus it was that I discovered the joy of skips.

I became a skip addict.* I was unable to pass one by without having a rummage to see what was being discarded. Bits of timber, panes of glass, old window

---

* For the benefit of my approximately three North American readers, a skip is, I believe, what you would call a dumpster.

frames – I rarely went out for a walk with the dog without returning carrying some treasure.

One skip in particular was a rich seam. A house nearby was having a complete remodelling, including all-new windows. On Christmas Day we returned from a day with friends with me carrying a wonderful unexpected gift: two window frames complete with panes of double-glazing. It was the skip's Christmas present to my shed.

Over the course of the rebuilding, I scavenged the following goodies, either from skips, or from the recycling bins down the bottom of the road:

Four double-glazed windows, complete with glass
Two extra pieces of double-glazed glass
Four pallets
An enormous piece of plywood
Two large pieces of chipboard
About ten metres of skirting board
About fifteen variously sized lengths of beading, moulding and other decorative woodwork
Two long pieces of guttering and some downpipe
A huge carpet
A digital radio (works perfectly)
A table
A lampstand
A lantern for the outside of the shed

I found skip-raiding an interesting experience. Generally I ask before taking, but in many cases the people aren't there to ask; the houses are dark, the workmen absent – off on other jobs – so I've just nabbed stuff. And often the skip was gone the next day anyway.

When you are walking home with a large lump of carpet that you have liberated from a skip, you feel both the thrill of discovery and a kind of shame that you have become the type of person who takes stuff from skips. At least, I felt that at first. I started by raiding the skips at night. I felt self-conscious about being seen poking around in skips, let alone carrying stuff away. But as time went by I kind of stopped caring.

I was doing a good thing, after all. I was recycling. Let them think what they want.

Mr Nobody

Who are you? You, my friend, are somebody. But I have this to tell you: in order to know who that somebody is, you have to become a nobody first. Yes, I know. It's suddenly gone all Karate Kid. Zen lite. But it's true. It's a biblical principle that in order to become somebody you have to become a nobody. Jacob was a wealthy and successful man, but in the river he was stripped of everything that previously gave him identity. And it is in that moment that God gives him a new name.

The same is true of many biblical characters. Jacob's son Joseph goes through a similar journey – left for dead, sold into slavery, ending up in an Egyptian prison. Moses loses his status as an Egyptian prince and becomes an outcast working as a shepherd in the desert. Much later, Paul loses all his carefully garnered religious clubcard points on the road outside Damascus and is left completely helpless. Later he included in one of his letters an early church hymn which set out how Jesus, too, gave up everything in order to become human, how he 'emptied himself, taking the form of a slave, being born in human likeness' (Philippians 2:7).

When Jacob thinks he is winning the fight, he demands a blessing. But it is only when he is beaten and humbled and limping that he receives a gift from God: a new name and a new identity. And part of that identity is humility.

We see this played out in what happens next. One would think, given what he has been through, that when Jacob met Esau the next day, he would be proud of his achievement. After all, he wrestled God and survived! But instead he treats Esau with the utmost deference. He bows seven times as he approaches. He calls Esau 'my lord' and describes himself as Esau's servant. He says to his brother, 'truly to see your face is like seeing the face of God – since you have received me with such favour'.

What has happened to this man? Simple. He is under new management. He has a new status and a new power, and that is why, in his encounter with Esau, he doesn't need to worry about any power or status of his own. He has touched God, wrestled with God, been blessed by God. Now he is renamed and ruled by God. Indeed, although Genesis links the name Israel to Jacob's struggle with God, it can also mean 'God rules' or 'God protects'. Up until this point in Jacob's life, Jacob might well have been called *israjacob* – 'Jacob rules'. Now God is in charge.[45]

Down to earth

I am trying a new discipline these days, a very difficult discipline for me. I am going into shops and asking for assistance. This is extremely hard for men like me: first, because I don't like to get into any conversation with shop assistants in case I have to buy something out of politeness, and second, because, well, I'm a hunter-gatherer. What kind of hunter-gatherer is it who has to ask for directions? *'Excuse me, the thing is, I need some new arrows for my bow, you know, to go mammoth hunting and all that. Yes, I know that normally we make the arrows ourselves, but you know, I just thought maybe buying them might be easier . . .'*

But it's so tiring, pretending all the time that you can do things all on your own, that you don't need help. And anyway, middle age will bring humility, whether we like it or not. As a middle-aged man I find there are more than enough factors to keep me humble. We age, we decline, we slow down, we're sidelined, we're past our sell-by date, we're obsolete – you know, who cares, I mean, really, *who cares*? The burden of worrying about what others think of us can be a crushing weight.

---

* I haven't started asking for directions, though. There are some things that a man should never do.

To put aside our pride and our need for status is liberating. I've carried them long enough. I'm ready to find out who I am.

Honesty brings humility. To see ourselves as we are, to recognise our own failings, fears and false identities is a humbling thing. But that's OK, because for Christians, humility is the aim of maturity. And humility is the gateway to a more fulfilling life.

Humility always shocks people. Our post-Darwinian dog-eat-dog society is all about looking out for number one. 'It's a jungle out there, son, and only the big beasts survive.' We need a better perspective. So, three things to learn.

First lesson: being humble is not the same as being humiliated. Humility is not about self-hatred or self-abuse. Humility is fundamentally having a proper view of yourself and your purpose. Anthony Bloom writes:

> The word 'humility' comes from the Latin word *humus* which means fertile ground ... Humility is the situation of the earth. The earth is always there, always taken for granted, never remembered, always trodden on by everyone, somewhere we cast and pour out all the refuse, all we don't need. It's there, silent and accepting everything and in a miraculous way making out of all the refuse new richness in spite of corruption, transforming corruption itself into a power of new life and a new possibility of creativeness . . .[46]

Humility is liberating. Because once we gain true humility we are free from worrying about what other people think of us. I'm going to talk more about this in a while, but for the moment, here's the summary: for heaven's sake, let's not take ourselves so seriously. Trevor Hudson talks of the 'everyday humiliations of the false self' – the embarrassing things which life brings our way to remind ourselves of who we really are. And the thing is that it's the *false self* which is affected by these events, that polished but so superficial exterior which we arrange neatly to present to the world. The false self has to be tripped up, has to fall flat on its arse occasionally, because otherwise we might start to believe our own publicity.

Really holy men aren't afraid to look foolish. As one of the Desert Fathers said, 'Do not expect your words to be taken seriously when you speak, and you will find peace.'[47]

Humility does not mean thinking that I don't matter, but recognising that I don't *need* to matter, at least only to certain people. Look, I think we can all agree that I have been scandalously overlooked for the Booker Prize, the Costa, the Whitbread, the Nobel Prize for literature and the Horse of the Year Show. But I can't control that. And I am tired of caring so much about what people think. It matters to me what my wife and family think of me. It matters to me what my friends think of me. Most of all, it matters to me what God thinks of me. Beyond that, I really don't have much control. All I have to concern myself with is acting with honesty and courage, and living out a life that reflects my deepest values. In the words of Dallas Willard, 'If our lives and works are to be of the Kingdom of God we must not have human approval as a primary or even major aim. We must lovingly allow people to think what they will.'[48]

Don't get me wrong. I don't want people to think badly

of me. Contrary to popular opinion, I don't set out to annoy people, and I don't enjoy it when I say or write things that turn out to upset people. But I can't be thinking of that when I start to type. I have to think of what God wants me to say, as best as I can discern it.

So, stop worrying about what people think of you. There is nothing worse than a middle-aged man trying to be cool. You were never cool anyway. There are only three really cool people on the planet, and they are Johnny Depp, Tom Waits and Pope Francis, and we can't compete with them. Allow yourself to feel things. Get rid of any self-imposed restrictions on showing emotion. Tell people you love them. Cry during movies. Have *fun*.

Second lesson of humility: understand that you are very small. What would spring to mind if I asked you to recount a humbling experience? Maybe you would tell me of some embarrassment, one of those humiliations of the false self. Or maybe you would talk of being somewhere really vast and feeling very small, one of those 'numinous' experiences at the top of a mountain, or in the face of a storm. Someone said to me the other day that the easy cure for pride is simply to go outside and lie down and look up at the stars for twenty minutes.*

This was Jacob's experience. At the end of his fight he was in a state of awe. 'I have seen God face to face,' he says, 'and yet my life is preserved' (Genesis 32:30). The word 'numinous' comes from the Latin *numen*, meaning 'a divine being'. The word was first coined by Rudolph Otto in his book *The Idea of the Holy*. A numinous

---

* Do this in summer, though. If you do it in winter, you might cure your pride, but you will then need a cure for hypothermia.

experience creates awe, fear and feelings of what he called our 'creatureliness'. God, he said, was the *numinosum* – the source of numinousness. Er . . . numinosity.[49] Anyway, a numinous experience comes about when we feel in touch with some deep spiritual power, and often this occurs in places where we get a sense of proper perspective: mountaintops, islands, what the Celts called 'thin' places. After the fight Jacob raised a cairn to mark the place; maybe in future years people passing by sensed that feeling: we are very small people in a very big world.

Which brings us to the third lesson of humility: realise how powerless you are. Jacob discovered this. He thought he was doing really well in the wrestling match and then, with a flick of a hand, he was hit with the mother of all groin injuries. Jacob was a strong man capable of moving a big stone, and he gave a good account of himself, but in the end his opponent simply reached out and touched him, and that was that. Game over.*

We are, in the end, pretty powerless in these dark night struggles. But that's OK. Christianity dares to proclaim the power of weakness. In one of its most powerful (albeit slightly weird) pictures of Jesus, he is seen as a dead lamb. Paul proudly claims that it is in his weakness that God is most powerfully present.

Addicts get this. In AA groups members admit their

---

* The Hebrew word means 'hollow of his thigh'. It seems to indicate the hip socket. The story says that this is why Jews do not eat the muscle of the thigh bone. But strangely nothing is said in the remainder of the Old Testament about this practice. So no one knows why that is there.

own powerlessness and they work at understanding it together. Humility pushes us into the arms of others. In quest stories the hero needs the help of others – and often he has to learn that the hard way. You need companions to get you through the dark places – the deserts, the forests, the Odyssey-style *nekyia*, the storm. This can be difficult, because so many men struggle along without any intimate friends, feeling alone and trapped.

I think a lot of men feel isolated. We have many mates, but few friends. We need proper friends. Facebook friends, just to be clear, are not friends. The blokes down the pub are not friends. The dog is described as man's best friend, and, though I love my dog, I wouldn't trust him for advice. Real friends are those with whom we can share our honest understanding of ourselves and who, in turn, will bring us the saving word. They are those who will help us to make decisions, tell us when we're being stupid, or sometimes just enjoy being stupid with us. They are the people with whom we can be honest. It can be difficult for men to talk about things like fear and anxiety. We've been trained to be strong, to be in control. Stress is for wimps, fear is for failures. It's hard to find the language to allow us to talk of things we are not supposed to feel in the first place.

To be humble is to realise that I am not in charge. I have to learn to let go. The German word for serenity is *Gelassenheit*, which literally means 'having let go'.[50]

The first half of life may be driven by acquisition, but the second half is powered by relinquishment. I need to let go of my need to be right, to be in control, to be safe. When we let go of these things, our work, our failures, our possessions, our masks, it does not mean that we do without them or that we dismiss them completely. It means that we view them in a proper perspective.

Humility willingly chosen is transformative and liberating – it is the key to progress. Once we recognise that we can do nothing, really, in our own power, then we can turn to the real source of power with which to move forward.

Earlier I talked about sin being a movement away from God. When we start to address our sin, what we are really doing is turning around. The Bible has a word for this, and it is 'repentance'. It's another word which has come to be loaded with all kinds of false associations, normally of miserable sinners on their knees, weeping and wailing and flagellating themselves. Or perhaps it is a perfunctory box-ticking exercise where we confess our sins, mutter 'sorry' like a boy dragged in front of the headmaster, and move quickly on.

That is not repentance. The word means much more than that. The Greek word *metanoeo* means 'to turn around', 'to undergo a change in frame of mind and feeling, to make a change of principle and practice, to reform'. It means changing not only our minds, but our behaviour, a 'decision by the whole man to turn round'.[51]

I introduce this now because I want to get a key point across. What I have tried to stress is that we need to reject the false gods and embrace the real one. But that raises a real question for many men. We may be keen to leave all the rubbish stuff behind, but that doesn't mean we are at all convinced that God would welcome us.

We might want to embrace the real God, but what if he doesn't want to embrace us?

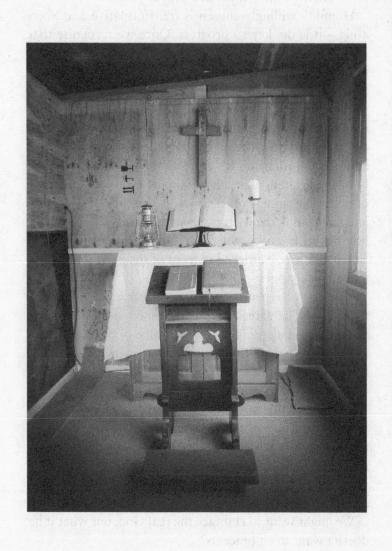

6

EMBRACING

Church building

I was about halfway through rebuilding when I realised that the project had changed.

The new windows were in. The walls were back up and insulated. The roof was still leaking a bit ... As I had gone along I had mostly worked around the contents of the shed. But finally I was ready to put the carpet down – the carpet that I'd 'rescued' from another skip round the corner. And once I put the carpet down, I realised that I quite liked the shed left empty. In other words, I wasn't sure whether what I wanted was really a 'shed' at all.

Maybe it was the door that did it. I'd taken a piece of coloured glass out of an old front door and built it into the shed door. It gave a rather church-like feel to the entrance, like stained glass.

Actually, looking back, it was the book's fault. Either as an attempt to encourage me, or as a reminder of just how sad I actually was, The Wife had bought me another shed book: a copy of Gordon Thorburn's *Men and Sheds*, a collection of black-and-white photos of men and, unsurprisingly, given the title, their sheds. 'The fascinating story of each man and his shed is accompanied by revealing photographs of both the customised exterior and the inner sanctum,' ran the blurb on the back. The author, it promised, 'delves into the sheds of British blokes to discover the personalities and passions hidden within it, be it a workshop crammed with strange inventions, a chapel, the home of a milk bottle collection, an allotment shed . . .'[52] Wait a minute. A chapel? A *chapel*?

There it was. Page 50. An unnamed suffragan bishop standing in his shed in his full bishopy costume. The building had bare walls, a spindle-legged table with a Bible on it, three candles, and a crucifix the size of a small car. Not quite to my taste, and with a shameful lack of double glazing (he said smugly), but a chapel, and one in which a record congregation of sixteen had gathered at one time.

No room for sixteen in mine. Three, maybe. But a seed was planted. Previously the shed had contained a big sideboard which held all the old tools and bits and pieces. I cut that down and turned it into a single chest of drawers. The entire previous contents of the shed were whittled down to as little as possible.

On the back wall I put an old cupboard door – another remnant of the girls' toy cupboard – on which I started to pin prayer requests and things to remember. The door is a reminder to ask: 'Knock and it shall be given to you.'

Then, at the end of the shed I put the cupboard – the one made out of that old dresser. I covered it with a piece of white hessian. On the top I placed a paraffin lamp and a cast-iron cookery book holder, on which I put a Bible. I fashioned a candlestick out of an old table lamp and a piece of Bakelite. And on the wall above it a crudely knocked-together cross, made of two pieces of two-by-one wood.

The final touch was discovered while visiting friends on

the south coast. We found an old prayer desk on the pavement outside an antique shop. A prie-dieu, made of dark oak, with a thin, sloping shelf for a prayer book and a board to kneel on, which was padded with what looked suspiciously like carpet underlay.

'You need that for your shed,' said The Wife.

She was right. It was no longer a workplace, a place to fashion either wood or words. Or at least it was those things, but it was more.

I set out to rebuild a shed, but along the way it turned into a chapel.

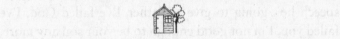

The wrong story

In one of his most famous stories, Jesus told a tale about two sons and their father. One day the youngest son makes a scandalous request. He wants to have his inheritance money up front, i.e. without having to wait for his dad to do all that tedious 'dying' bit. Amazingly, the old man agrees. So the younger son takes his share of the property and goes off with his stash and basically squanders it all on what the King James Version called 'riotous living'. (Later we find out that it involves call girls. I think we can also assume alcohol.) Anyway, he spends the lot and ends up in the gutter, deserted and utterly destitute. He is reduced to working with pigs – which for a Jewish boy was the lowest of the low. He is so hungry that he tries to eat the pig food. Eventually he comes to his senses and realises that he has made a hash of his life and that he should go home and just work as a slave for his dad, where even the lowest, most menial worker is looked after better than he is.

So he trudges home, in his filthy, mud-spattered, pigshit-ruined clothes. You can imagine the shame as he walks back through his home village. The finger-pointing and the laughter and all the parents preparing an Improving Moral Lesson for their children. Maybe he's avoiding their eye, maybe he doesn't even notice. After all, he's gone beyond that now, he's well below the sea-level of shame. All he's doing the whole way is rehearsing the speech he's going to give – 'Father, I've failed God, I've failed you, I'm not good enough to be your son any more, but please, just *please* give me a job.'

And he's concentrating on this speech so hard that he never even sees the old man coming. Maybe at the last moment he catches something out of the corner of his downcast eye, maybe he hears the dry slap of rapid footsteps and the wheezy old man's breathing, but then – WHAM – the old man hits him like a steam train, wraps him up in the biggest bear hug ever. It's half-hug, half-rugby tackle. And the son tries to deliver his speech, but he can't even get his words out, because the old man is laughing and whooping and crying all at once. Apparently he had been out most days, staring into the distance, watching eagerly for his son to come home. And he's so happy that this has happened, so overjoyed that his son has returned, that he throws a party. Of course, when the older brother hears that sonny-boy is home he gets really upset. He had stayed home and done his duty and he never got so much as a Christmas cracker. But the old man insists that they have to rejoice. 'Your brother was dead,' he says, probably still wheezing from his sprint earlier in the day, 'but now he's come back to life. He was lost and now he's found.'

It's called the story of the prodigal son. That's 'prodigal' as in 'recklessly wasteful, extravagant, profligate, improvident, imprudent'. But it should be the story of the prodigal father. Because if anyone is recklessly wasteful, extravagant, profligate, improvident and imprudent, it's him.

Considering the time the story was told, it's a truly astonishing picture of God. A culture that saw God as the ultimate arbiter, the great law-giver on high, is shown instead a God who runs down the road and welcomes back his returning son with a party. Never mind dignity, never mind finger-wagging: this God is a joyous, forgiving, loving God with a considerable turn of speed.

We turn back towards God, but he runs towards us so fast we barely see him coming.

The right story

One of the most unusual aspects of Jesus' teaching was his view of God. In the stories Jesus tells about God, he is presented as a lavishly, foolishly over-generous father, a rather daft shepherd who cares so much about just one sheep that he rushes off and leaves the other ninety-nine, a carelessly imprudent ruler who forgives tens of thousands of pounds of debt, a ruler who trusts his servants with untold riches, and an employer who pays a day's rate to the least regarded workers who only worked for an hour! There are times when he is stern, of course, but this tends to be when the lavish, risky generosity that he models is not replicated by others. This is a God who loves people but hates it when they don't pass it on.

Jesus himself lived this out as well. The Gospels portray him as a party-goer, a man who ate and drank with the wrong sort of people, who provided ready meals when people were hungry and turned the sterile water used for religious rituals into fine wine for a wedding party. It's like opening up the baptismal font to find it full of champagne. Indeed, one of the predominant pictures of Jesus in the Gospels is of a man who cares little for religious convention. In the binary world of first-century Judaism, everything was either clean or unclean: there were pure people and impure people. And Jesus kept spending his time with the wrong sort.

Like his father, he has his flashpoints: he can't stand religious humbug, hates the way that outcasts are treated, and refuses to treat those in authority with anything approaching respect. He is particularly hard on hypocrites. The Greek word *hupokrites* means 'actor'. In Greek and Roman theatre the actors all wore masks – and the Latin word for that mask was *persona*. Given all the Jung stuff, it should give us pause for thought that the behaviour which draws the most condemnation from Jesus is when people pretend to be one thing, but are something quite different in reality.

As well as telling stories which completely recalibrated what people thought they knew about God, Jesus' teaching was similarly mind-warping:

Do you love your friends? Anyone can do that. I say you have to love your enemies.

Give to those who ask, spend your love lavishly, do not return violence for violence.

You have to be forgiven – and you must forgive others.

Above all else, Jesus was himself. He had no airs and graces. Even the term he used for himself – 'Son of Man' – drew on the Aramaic term for 'ordinary bloke'.[53] People said of his teaching that he spoke 'like someone with authority'. In other words, he didn't bother piling up lots of justifications and precedents and proofs for what he said. He just *said* stuff. And people responded. They found something compelling about him. He drew people like a magnet – both the respectably religious and the disreputable 'sinners'. People left their jobs and their homes to become his disciples – his apprentices, trainees. Notorious sinners made outrageous public demonstrations of gratitude and commitment.

Why? Because they saw someone who could offer them the chance of a new life. That is exactly what he promised his followers, in fact: a life that meant something. He said that he had come to bring them life in all its fullness. But it would cost those who followed him everything. Paradoxically, real life can cost you your life.

It certainly cost him *his* life. On his final trip up to Jerusalem he was arrested by the cabal in charge of the temple, handed over to the Romans in a bit of political horse-trading, beaten savagely, tortured and finally crucified – a death the Romans reserved for slaves or foreign insurrectionaries.

And that was that. Except for the fact that three days later the tomb which held him was empty. And his followers started to claim that they had seen him. First the women at the tomb. Then some of his key followers. Then family members. In fact, one of his later followers, a man who had his own mid-life crisis, claimed that over five hundred people had seen Jesus at one time.

And his followers started to work out what it was all about. And what it meant – *part* of what it all meant – was that on that cross, Jesus had taken onto himself all the bad stuff of humanity, all the broken, soiled, shameful things which we've done, the petty misdemeanours and the great crimes, all the darkness and delusions and despair. He took all that the world could throw at him and held on to it so hard that he took it down with him. All the loneliness and fear, all the pain and the hatred, all the greed and selfishness. He wrapped it in his arms in a great cosmic wrestling hold and took it down into submission, took it with him into death.

And all that stuff died. But Jesus came back.

The story of Jesus is one of radical love and wild hope. And this is why it is so important. Because it is the ultimate expression of a promise which is woven into the very heart of humanity, the promise of resurrection, the promise that we can start again. And if there's one thing all of us need, it's a spot of resurrection.

Are these the stories we hear (or tell) about God and Jesus, though? I wonder. Often, I think we are told very different stories. God is an old bloke with a beard. Distant, aloof and with no discernible sense of humour, he is only really interested in us if we grovel. His son, meanwhile, is a long-haired, pale-skinned creature, given to wandering about Galilee wearing a nightie and looking all mystical. Even the church – *especially* the church – often reinforces these pictures. All the old songs about God are full of big words. He is immortal, invisible, ineffable (whatever that means), while many modern songs about Jesus make it sound as though he's a girl we're trying to get off with. And preachers manage to make both of them sound like the most boring beings imaginable.

Everything depends on these stories. How much we desire to turn towards God and to seek to follow Jesus is entirely dependent on the stories we tell and the stories we are told about them. If we have a false narrative about God, we will not want to return to him, no matter how much pigswill we have consumed. How we view God affects our ability and our desire to change. It affects how you and I think about ourselves and whether we actually want to go anywhere near his kingdom.

Let's face it, our view of God affects absolutely *everything*.

Pictures of God

How did Jacob view God, I wonder? At one point, after all, his father Isaac had been on the point of being sacrificed to God, given up as a burnt offering, before God spared Abraham's son – and Abraham – at the last minute. Perhaps it's not so surprising that Isaac's relationship with God is somewhat distant. Of all the patriarchs, he has the least direct communion with God. Perhaps Jacob was affected by his father's view of God. Perhaps that's the reason why he does so much for himself, and why he tries to tie God into a deal. Maybe he never fully trusted the God his father had told him about.

There are many false narratives about God. Certainly my image of God was of someone who was, overall, a bit disappointed in me. He was the 'I'm not angry, just very disappointed' God – who really hoped that I would turn out better and who just sighs and shakes his head whenever I do another dumb thing. At times he is so let down by me that he becomes the 'unavailable' God. I am told he is there, but he won't take my calls. There is nothing but endless ringing, or an angel putting me on hold.

Then there is the 'passive-aggressive God', the one who says, 'Of course I forgive you. I'm fine. No, really.' And then he goes and does a load of sneaky things behind our backs to ruin our lives, while all the time pretending to be over it. And when we challenge him, say to him, 'This is all about that lust thing, isn't it?' he replies, 'What? No! How can you say that? I'm God, for my sake. I don't do that kind of thing.'

Or you get the 'God of wrath', who has given up on head-shaking and tutting, and is actively sharpening up the thunderbolts. At his worst, he becomes 'Bronze-age War-crazed Shock-and-awe God', who appears occasionally in the Bible (mainly in Joshua). We don't like to talk about him, generally. He swallows our prayers and worship like Prozac. They just about serve to keep him calm. Most of the time he really, really wants to smite us, but Jesus keeps talking him out of it.

Equally false, at the other end of the spectrum there is the 'Everything's lovely and just be nice' God: the divine equivalent of My Little Pony, all pink and fluffy and never angry about anything. So don't worry about bad stuff and suffering and evil and justice, because everything is sunny and, you know, just marshmallows.

And then there is the loneliest God of all. The non-existent God. The one who isn't there, and whose absence leaves a gaping, meaningless hole at the heart of everything.

So many false narratives about God.

It's a curious thing, but our false narratives about God spring from false narratives about ourselves. We think of ourselves primarily as sinners, so we view God as wrathful; we feel small, lost and lonely, so we think God is absent or non-existent; we hate ourselves and our failings, so we imagine that God will never return our calls.

Because we ourselves find so much of what we do unforgivable, we think that we can never be forgiven. Because we do not accept ourselves, we do not think that God can accept us. He might tolerate us, put up with us for those brief moments in between sins, but he doesn't really *love* us. No one could see all the things we do, and hear all the thoughts we think, and still love us. So we turn the story on its head and think that, although God welcomes back repentant sinners, he really prefers the elder son type, the ones who stay at home and never cause trouble. He takes us back, because it's in the job description. He is contractually obliged to forgive. There may be a job for us with the hired hands, but there will be no parties.

Even great men have had difficulty in accepting that God loves them. Henri Nouwen wrote,

Can I accept that I am worth looking for? Do I believe that there is a real desire in God to simply be with me?

Here lies the core of my spiritual struggle: the struggle against self-rejection, self-contempt, and self-loathing. It is a very fierce struggle because the world and its demons conspire to make me think about myself as worthless, useless, and negligible.[54]

Well, the good thing is that God is big enough to deal with our false narratives about him. He is big enough to deal with honesty.

Later on I will look at some exercises we can do to deepen our understanding of God and to challenge our own false narratives. But for the moment I want to concentrate on two main things, things which have taken me most of my life to understand, and which, having at last grasped, I am only now starting to explore. These two things are that God loves us, and he is with us. Right here, right now.

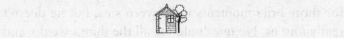

Bidden or not bidden

Bidden or not bidden, God is there. Funny how stuff crops up once and then pops up again and again. You start to spot it everywhere. At a retreat, a friend of mine showed me a plaque on which was a phrase which had deeply affected her: *Bidden or not bidden, God is there.* She had been so struck by this statement that she had actually bought the plaque – and this is a woman who does not even own her own sofa. A week later I was at another event where the speaker said the very same thing. So I thought maybe God was trying to say something and I looked up where it came from. It led back to our friend Jung.

Jung had the phrase – in Latin – inscribed over the doorway of his house, and upon his tomb. He put the inscription there 'to remind my patients and myself: *Timor dei initium sapiente*'. Which means, 'the fear of the Lord is the beginning of wisdom'. The inspiration wasn't original to Jung – it originally comes from ancient Greece, from the Delphic Oracle, the people who brought you 'Know Yourself'. In the fifth century BC the Spartans were about to go to war with the Athenians, and they sent a message asking the oracle for guidance. According to Thucydides, 'The god replied that if they fought with all their might, victory would be theirs, and that he himself would be on their side, *whether they invoked him or not.*'[55] Say what you like about the Delphic Oracle, he/she/it produced some great material. I can imagine the Spartans put this on their T-shirts and badges – along with 'We are Sparta!' and 'I ♥ proto-fascist States'.

Whatever its origins, it contains a deep truth. Called or uncalled, bidden or unbidden, God is present. And what was good enough for Carl was good enough for me. Twenty years ago, I did a woodcarving course, after which I'd bought a piece of pale cherry wood, intending to carve my masterpiece. Nothing happened, and the wood had sat in the shed ever since. In the clearout I rediscovered it, forlorn and forgotten at the back of an old cupboard. I planed it smooth(ish), cleaned up my old chisels, carved some rough letters and inked them in.

The sign went up in the shed soon after.

Bidden or not bidden, God is there.

Closer than you know

In the dark night of the soul we search for God, and find only his absence. He seems remote, fugitive. But God is not distant, nor absent; he is closer than we can possibly imagine. And the reason we can't see him is because he is actually enveloping us. We can't see him because he is simply too big, too close, too present. He is all around us, above and below and within.

God is there. God is *always* there.

God, says the Bible, is the very grounds of our being. In that sense, of course, we can never turn back to God, we can only recognise his presence. But I guess that amounts to the same thing. Anyway, God is everywhere and in all:

> *Where can I go from your spirit?*
> *Or where can I flee from your presence?*
> *If I ascend to heaven, you are there;*
> *if I make my bed in Sheol, you are there.*
>
> (Psalm 139:7-8)

He was with us before we were even aware of him. God tells Jeremiah:

> *Before I formed you in the womb I knew you,*

and before you were born I consecrated you;
I appointed you a prophet to the nations.

(Jeremiah 1:5)

Paul could confidently tell a group of Athenian wannabe philosophers that in God 'we live and move and have our being' (Acts 17:28).

Post-biblical writers took up this theme. Augustine spent a life searching for God, only to find him closer than he thought: 'And see, you were within and I was in the external world and sought you there, and in my unlovely state I plunged into these lovely created things which you made. You were with me and I was not with you . . .'[56]

The medieval book known as *The Cloud of Unknowing*[*] says that 'God is your being, and what you are, you are in God'.[57]

One of the key things to understand if we are ever going to crawl out from under this mid-life rock is that we are not alone. I know, it *feels* that way. In the dark night it feels like we have been deserted, separated, that we are standing there at midnight in the freezing cold river, watching all we have ever striven for and cared for in life moving away into the distance. But we are not alone. How could we be? As Martin Laird says in his brilliant book *Into the Silent Land*, 'Because God is the ground of our being, the relationship between creature and Creator is such that, by sheer grace, separation is not possible. God does not know how to be absent.'[58]

---

[*] In keeping with its title, we don't know who the author is. Probably a Carthusian monk.

Jesus used the image of the vine to describe his relationship with his followers: 'I am the vine, you are the branches. Those who abide in me and I in them bear much fruit, because apart from me you can do nothing' (John 15:5). We are branches, twigs, always part of the vine. 'A branch doesn't seek the vine; it's already part of the vine,' says Martin Laird. 'A wave doesn't look for the ocean; it's already full of ocean.'

Bidden or unbidden, God is there.

We are a wave on the ocean. We are a branch of the vine.

Or, perhaps, a leaf on an oak tree.

The God who wrestles

I talked about the punning nature of Jacob's tale. The river Jabbok – *yabbok* – is close to the Hebrew word for 'wrestling', *yeabeq*. But it's also close to another Hebrew word: *habaq* – which means 'an embrace'.

In London, with time to kill before a meeting, I wandered into Tate Britain. Turning a corner, I came across an enormous statue. Carved out of brown and cream marble, two huge figures stand face to face. One of them has massive, slab wings on his back. He is an angel, and he is crouching down so that he is face to face with the other figure – if he stood he would be head and shoulders taller. Although clasped together, they are no longer fighting. Instead the angel is supporting the other figure, holding him tenderly, lifting him like a wounded man. His arms reach round, embracing him, supporting him, raising him up on tiptoe. The man he is holding lies back, slumped, semi-conscious, arms hanging limply by his side. He is utterly defeated.

The statue is *Jacob and the Angel*, by Jacob Epstein. I stood and gazed at it for a long time. It has since become an icon for me, a picture which leads me deeper into an experience of God. Capable of enormous power, this God chooses to lift us like a father lifting a toddler. God holds us and supports us. Raises us up. Enfolds us in his arms with a tender love. We thought it was a fight; turns out it was always a hug.

Jacob only understood this later, I think. At the time, he was literally fighting for his life; that is, for his life to have meaning. He fought to find out if there was something worth fighting for. He had lost everything. He had spent years misunderstanding God, but maybe something in him told him that the fight was still worth it. He had enough honesty and enough self-knowledge to revisit his narrative about God and believe that maybe things had got skewed along the way. That, instead of doing 'deals', God kept promises. That's why Jacob wrestled.

Why, though, did God wrestle? First, because that was what Jacob wanted and needed at that time. And second, because it was the only possible way for Jacob to finally become the person he was meant to be. And behind both reasons lay love.

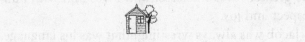

The humility of God

One of the amazing things in this story is that God was willing to get his hands dirty. In the Epstein sculpture in the Tate, the angel stoops to hold the beaten, broken Jacob. And that is what happened: God stooped to Jacob's level. He came down and had a fight. This is the Prodigal God in action, not a farmer at a gate this time, but a wrestler in a river.

Throughout the Bible we see the humility of God. God is willing to descend to our level in order to raise us up to his. His willingness to fight with Jacob is just one example of his willingness to be with any human in the way which is deepest and truest for them. With Jacob he was willing to wrestle. With Jacob's grandfather, Abraham, God was willing to be bargained with. With their distant descendant Moses, he was willing to be argued with. Each man meets with God in the way that suits him best, and the way which will change him most profoundly.

John of the Cross recognised this. 'He loves thee with the greatest humility, and with the greatest esteem,' he said of God, 'making thee His equal, joyfully revealing Himself to thee, in these ways.'[59] For most ancient cultures, this kind of friendship would have been unthinkable. In Aristotle's view, friendship was possible only from the lesser to the greater, or among equals. But here we have the upside-down world of God, whereby the greater loves the lesser and loves him with humility, respect and joy.

Jacob was always wrestling: that was his language. The very first form of communication Jacob learnt was a fight.

The story tells how, even before they were born, the twins fought, having a punch-up in their mother's womb. The antenatal fighting got so bad that Rebekah despaired: 'The children struggled together within her; and she said, "If it is to be this way, why do I live?"' (Genesis 25:22) She didn't need a scan to find out what life was going to be like. But years later, God uses this base language of violence to change Jacob.

God uses our deepest, core 'languages' to speak to us: our innate feelings, the things to which we respond at the deepest level. Is that music? Art? Sport? Mountain climbing? Græco-Roman wrestling? It differs for each of us, but I believe that God speaks to each as he needs, and in the way he will understand.

For some of us, like Jacob, God uses our dreams. I dream every night. Every. Single. Night.* I'm not going to tell you my dreams here, because (a) other people's dreams are pretty boring, and (b) mine are so bizarre that you might lose what little faith you have remaining in my wisdom. But I have learnt that my dreams can be a source of insight, or a source of strength. Sometimes they are your standard-issue anxiety dreams – which in my case are generally about trying to get somewhere on the train with enormous amounts of luggage – but at other times they provide me with images which, on reflection, can be sources of strength. Most of the time, of course, they are merely sources of amusement for The Wife.† But listen to

---

* Actually, everybody dreams, apparently. It's just that not everyone remembers their dreams.
† I once met a woman who had just done a course in dream interpretation and was confident of her ability to interpret the

your dreams. Look for the ways in which God may be speaking to you.

God in his mercy thought it a good use of his time to fight with this man. God respects Jacob, values him, believes Jacob to be worth the struggle. Why? Because Jacob still hadn't become the person God intended him to be.

The best a man can get

God wrestled with Jacob because it was the only way for Jacob to turn into the person God intended him to be. That is God's ambition for us: to flourish as the person he created, to grow into the person he always meant us to be.

For years I thought that one of the reasons I was a failure was that I was not someone else. I thought that in order for God to accept me, I would have to change into another person entirely. Maybe become a monk. And I found this depressing. I mean, I had nothing against monks, I even had the hairstyle, albeit by accident, and I had certainly embraced a monk-like poverty, but I didn't want to be a monk. Nonetheless, I was convinced that the current model of 'Nick Page' was never going to make the

obscurest images. I told her the one where Sir Tom Jones taught me his special London parking method, which basically involved parking his Rolls-Royce vertically, in a hole in the road. She looked at me and said, 'Er . . . they haven't covered that one on the course yet.'

grade. I used to look at people I admired, wise and warm and holy people, and think, 'I need to turn into them.' And so I would try on their persona for a bit – but the mask kept slipping. Whatever shape I tried to adopt, I couldn't help but revert to the same old Nick Page-shaped failure.

Eventually, I realised that you can never become who God wants you to be if you are ashamed of who you are. God doesn't want me to be someone else: he wants me to be Nick Page. He created Nick Page, with all his joys and pains and passions and stupidities. He specifically designed an experiment to see what the world would look like with a Nick Page in it. And God can't wait to see how I turn out.

I love my children, but that doesn't mean that I want to keep them as children for the rest of their lives. I loved them as toddlers, but I was really pleased when they stopped needing nappies. What my love for them means is that I want them to become whole and complete individuals, capable of loving God, loving themselves and loving their neighbour. I want the best for them – above all, that they should grow up to fulfil their potential in relationship with God. That is what love means. I don't want them to be other people. I want them to be truly, happily, wholly themselves.

Think about those we love. We love them for who they are. We wouldn't want them to be someone else. I love The Wife because of who she is. And I wake up every day wondering how much more herself she is going to be. It's a white-knuckle ride, I tell you. But I wouldn't want it any other way.

This is our old friend individuation. Individuation, as you may recall, is the process through which people become whole. The oak tree is the individuated version of the acorn. The chicken is an individuated egg. And no two are identical. Each is a 'complete *and* unique expression of life'.[60] You are unique. There is no one else exactly like you and there never will be. So the heart of our calling is to become the absolute best version of ourselves: the version that God had in mind when he was drawing up the plans.

And he *was* drawing up the plans. In the words of Psalm 139, God knit us together in our mother's womb.

> *My frame was not hidden from you,*
> *when I was being made in secret,*
> *intricately woven in the depths of the earth.*
> *Your eyes beheld my unformed substance.*
> *In your book were written*
> *all the days that were formed for me,*
> *when none of them as yet existed.*
>
> (Psalm 139:15-16)

We've already seen Jesus explaining that God knows the number of hairs on our heads (an easier job with some of us than with others, admittedly). But the Bible is clear: God knows us intimately and has plans for all of us from the start.

We see this in the story of Jacob. Rebekah, in her pre-natal despair about the twins fighting inside her, has the wisdom to consult the Lord. And somehow – we are not told how it happens exactly – God tells her something very significant:

> And the LORD said to her,
> 'Two nations are in your womb,
> and two peoples born of you shall be divided;
> the one shall be stronger than the other,
> the elder shall serve the younger.'
>
> (Genesis 25:23)

So God already had journeys planned for them both. God knew what was going to happen and he knew what he wanted to happen. But what God needed, really needed, what he longed for, with all the yearning of a father staring out into the distance in the hope that his son might return home, was that Jacob would grow up into the person he was always intended to be.

God has a purpose for you and a purpose for me. Now this kind of phrase always rings alarm bells for me: I don't, in this case, mean the kind of thing you often hear – you know, 'God wants you to go to Africa/Outer Mongolia/the corner shop and buy me a Magnum', or 'God wants you to become a nurse/doctor/unicyclist'. I mean, God *might* want that, but I'm not going to get all specific. And, frankly, I think in most cases God doesn't mind what you do as long as it's something that does some good. People get very wound up about this kind of thing. I have met several men who are desperate to hear from God what he wants them to do with their life. And others who thought they knew – were certain that they knew – only to find that it all went pear-shaped. So I think we have to be very careful with the specifics.

The fact is that we already know what God wants us to do with our life. He wants us to *live*. He wants us to put away the masks and the pretending and be the person we were meant to be. Jung said, 'True personality is always a vocation.'[61] We are our own vocation. We are our own calling.

And if I can crack this, then, you never know, some bits of me might, indeed, look a bit monk-like. I am inspired by the stories of the Desert Fathers, those strange, extreme hermits who embraced a life of solitude and dedication in the deserts of Egypt, Palestine and Syria from the fourth century onwards. In their lives I see a raw, extreme holiness that is utterly unlike anything I could ever achieve. But in one story, Abba (i.e. Father) Macarius asks a hermit called Zacharias, 'What makes a monk?' Zacharias answers, 'As far as I can tell, abba, I think anyone who controls himself and makes himself content with just what he needs and no more is, indeed, a monk.'[62] Well, I think I could aim for that.

But what does that look like? I know what you're thinking. You're thinking, 'Nick, you're already a glorious angelic creature, how can you possibly be better?' Well, thank you, I understand your awe. But there is a template for us to follow. What our lives should look like, in their best, their very best version, is Jesus. As my friend Trevor Hudson said, 'What would your life look like if Jesus was living it?'

This is, I think, what it means to enter the second half of life. It means to live your life, but with added Jesus.

Turbo-charged

By early February the shed was sound and dry. Well, dry-ish. I mean, the roof leaked in the far corner, and when I looked round the back I could see that at the bottom some boards had become loose. I ignored them, obviously.

The carpet was down and the roof (mostly) insulated. I bought a paraffin lamp. And I invited a friend round to play. Well, I say 'play'. I mean, 'talk to me about some brainy stuff'. Steve, as I like to think of him, is a psychiatrist. We sat in the shed, had a cup of tea and he talked about men, middle age and minds.

'When you've got everything you wanted, the things we classically strive for – the good woman, the mortgage, the kids, the job, for some people making a difference in the world – when you've got all that, *then* what do you do? For some people they end up feeling like there's a bit of a hole in the middle. A hole that no amount of money and material and even relationships, in a certain sense, will fill.

'Some people have within them a sense of security. In the jargon, we call it a secure base. But other people don't have that, and it's a central human need. When you ask people about that – and I ask a lot of people about it in my work, because a lot of my patients don't have it – they use a lot of different words but they're all talking about the same thing, which is a kind of hole, an absence inside them, psychologically.'

'Is this absence more pronounced in middle age?'

'It's not all or nothing. A lot of people have a degree of

it. So when you're young and everything's exciting it can get masked. When you start a family it can be masked, but when you reach the stage we're talking about – when most of your responsibilities are discharged and the really hard climb is over and your health isn't in decline – you have some space suddenly to notice the lack.

'I'm in the business of trying to make people more peaceful. That's what we do. They come to us with this big hole and we try to, not fill it, but shrink it, make it more bearable. Quite often it does become more bearable in quite a palpable way. At the end of eighteen months' treatment we talk about some of the things they've written and experienced and the change is quite astounding.' He thought for a moment. 'It's not something I often see mirrored in churches.'

'Why is that?'

'Well, two possibilities. One, that being a disciple of Christ doesn't reliably change you, or it changes you in a less subtle and noticeable way than other things change you. I know people who on one measure are very godly and serving God passionately, and on the other hand, their character doesn't seem to be changing in a godly way at all. One doesn't want to judge, but that's the way it can look.'

'And the second possibility?'

'The second possibility is that most of us are getting discipleship wrong. That we're doing it wrong. This is what you say, isn't it? The call to discipleship is something more radical than most of us think, and the reason most of us aren't being transformed is that we're not really discipling. You know, we're just mucking about.'

I asked him about his patients. 'How does transformation work with them?'

'There are two elements. First, honest, consistent, very straightforward feedback over many, many months. Second, the development of responsible agency, by which I mean, you insert your agency between the impulse and action. We try to point out the patterns and say, "This is what's going wrong." Then we say, "It doesn't have to be like this. But we can't change it; you can, because you're the one doing it." Many people say, "I can't do it. I see red, it's like a red mist. I don't even remember it – therefore it's not my fault" – which is rubbish. We say, "Listen, it is you doing this. We're not going to blame you for it, we're going to give you the opportunity to change."'

I could see so many parallels between what Steve was talking about and issues of discipleship. I talked to him about presenting people with a different narrative of God – a God who offered forgiveness and the opportunity to change. 'What would it look like,' I wondered, 'if we did that kind of thing in church?'

'The programme I run? You could model a discipleship programme on it. You could do that. You could insert prayers and communion and devotional stuff and make sure people understood the nature of God as you're talking about it, and do the whole honest feedback and responsible agency thing . . .' He paused. 'I suppose what you'd have to say is that you'd get similar results . . . But turbo-charged.'

Selving

There are plenty of people in the Bible who have to make the hard journey through to selfhood. The apostle Paul started out as Saul-the-Christian-hunter, until Jesus took him literally into a dark night, dazzled him into darkness, blinding him on his journey to destroy the Christian cell in Damascus. Sometimes we have to lose sight of everything before we can see things clearly. Certainly for Paul, the rest of his life was a long, painful, glorious journey into being the person God had always meant him to be. His letters show how earnestly he pushed towards that goal. He is always aware of his own shortcomings but never, ever less than Paul of Tarsus, and yet he himself says this: 'I have been crucified with Christ; and it is no longer I who live, but it is Christ who lives in me. And the life I now live in the flesh I live by faith in the Son of God, who loved me and gave himself for me' (Galatians 2:19-20).*

Somehow, Christ lives in us, and yet we are still us. Our 'us-ness', my 'me-ness', will not be eclipsed by Christ's presence, it will be enhanced, amplified, made alive. No one expressed this better than Gerard Manley Hopkins. Strap yourself in, it's poetry time.

'As Kingfishers Catch Fire'

As kingfishers catch fire, dragonflies draw flame;
As tumbled over rim in roundy wells

* The next paragraph begins, 'You stupid Galatians': see what I mean about him always being truly himself?

Stones ring; like each tucked string tells, each hung bell's
Bow swung finds tongue to fling out broad its name;
Each mortal thing does one thing and the same:
Deals out that being indoors each one dwells;
Selves – goes itself; myself it speaks and spells,
Crying What I do is me: for that I came.

I say more: the just man justices;
Keeps grace: that keeps all his goings graces;
Acts in God's eye what in God's eye he is –
Christ – for Christ plays in ten thousand places,
Lovely in limbs, and lovely in eyes not his
To the Father through the features of men's faces.

Isn't that fantastic! (And if you don't think it's fantastic, read it again. Read it again and again and again until you get what this holy man was saying.) We are all here to *selve*, in Hopkins' wonderful phrase: to express our true inward reality. And more than that, though, for we are not mere stones, or dragonflies, or even glorious azure, lightning-quick kingfishers: more than that, we are to reflect the life of Christ, 'lovely in limbs and lovely in eyes not his'. We are born to be both truly ourselves and truly like Christ. That is our privilege and our destiny and our hope.

Well, that's the offer on the table. But we have to accept it. God does not suddenly wave his magic wand and turn you from an ugly duckling into a swan. You have to put in the hard yards out on the pond, doing the swimming lessons and restraining the urge to quack.

In John's Gospel, Jesus heals a man who had been ill for thirty-eight years. The man is lying by the pool of Bethzatha or Bethesda, supposedly a place of healing, provided you could get into the water while the pool was being miraculously stirred. Jesus sees the man lying there and asks him a curious question: 'Do you want to be made well?'

Well, duh. Who *wouldn't* want to be made well? The man misunderstands him: he thinks that he is being accused of not making an effort. He explains that he can't get to the pool in time, he has no one to help him and everyone beats him to it.

Jesus ignores his excuses. He just issues an instruction: get up. 'Stand up, take your mat and walk.' We are not told if the man hesitated, or if he looked scared, or bewildered, or if he laughed. All we're told is that he stood up, lifted up his mat, and set off (John 5:2-9).

But it's a deep and profound question: do you *want* to be made well? Do you *want* to live?

I talked above about wanting to be holy. 'Holy' has come to mean something unusual, something sacred. And it is, in a way. But the root of the word is Old English for 'healthy', as in the phrase, 'hale and hearty'. Holiness is, in reality, the ultimate in healthiness. Or maybe we can use a different word, and have a look at a different holy book. Here, for example, is one of the most important passages ever written about spiritual formation:

'Real isn't how you are made ... It's a thing that happens to you. When a child loves you for a long, long time, not just to play with, but REALLY loves you, then you become Real.'

'Does it hurt?' asked the Rabbit.

'Sometimes,' said the Skin Horse, for he was always truthful. 'When you are Real you don't mind being hurt ... It doesn't happen all at once ... You become. It takes a long time ... Generally, by the time you are Real, most of your hair has been loved off, and your eyes drop out and you get loose in the joints and very shabby. But these things don't matter at all, because once you are Real you can't be ugly, except to people who don't understand.'[63]

If you ask me, *The Velveteen Rabbit* should be top of the list for any course of spiritual reading.

But that is what we want, isn't it? To become *real*. To stop being fake. It is God's embrace, God's wrestling which achieves that. And if, in the process, most of our hair gets rubbed off and our stuffing falls out and we become rather shabby, then I, for one, think that is a price worth paying.

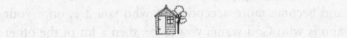

The art of not caring

Quick summary. So far I've argued this:

1. We experience a lot of bad stuff in mid-life. But that's good because ...
2. The crap we experience in mid-life is a call to whole-ness, and the great thing is that ...
3. Wholeness can be found in admitting our own failure and turning to God, which is nothing to be scared of because ...

4. God has been waiting all along for us to return to him because he loves us, and the amazing thing is ...

5. He wants us to become the person we were meant to be, the self who looks like Jesus.

When you grasp all this, slot it together piece by piece, it means *freedom*.

If we can *really* understand that God loves us, and wants us to become the real us, then we are liberated from the need to endlessly seek the approval of others. What we wear, the possessions we have, who is top dog, how many people report to us on the organisational chart – what does that matter, compared with whether or not I am becoming the person God wants me to be? As Dallas Willard said, 'We must lovingly allow people to think what they will.' [64]

Once you stop pretending to be something you're not and become more accepting of who you are, once your aim is who God wants you to be, then a lot of the other stuff doesn't seem to matter. (And the great thing about being a bit older is that you're *supposed* not to care about other people's opinion. You're expected to be a bit batty and eccentric. It's in the job description.)

Certainly, one of the characteristics of Jesus' life was his total independence.* He wasn't swayed by opinion or expectations. He refused to be the kind of Messiah that

---

* Jung saw individuation as giving people the power to live their own authentic life: 'And are not Jesus and Paul prototypes of those who, trusting their inner experience, have gone their own individual ways, disregarding public opinion?' (C.G. Jung, *The Undiscovered Self*, Signet Book, 2006, p. 57)

the Jews were expecting, i.e. a toff with a sword on a big horse who would drive out the Romans and make Israel Top Nation in perpetuity. At one point they wanted to make him king, and he ran away (John 6:15). He was often accused of breaking the Jewish religious law – actually, come to think of it, he was also accused of breaking Roman law. However, his impetus was always to live an authentic life of love. He never did it 'just because he could'. And while he did annoy a great many people in his life, I'm pretty sure he never set out to be annoying. It was just what happened when he loved people.

What matters is motive. When his followers were accused of breaking the Sabbath because they were foraging some food as they walked, Jesus said, 'The Son of Man is lord of the Sabbath.' In some ancient manuscripts there is a story of Jesus seeing a man working on the Sabbath day. 'Friend,' he says to him, 'if you know what you are doing you are blessed, but if you do not know, you are accursed as a breaker of the law.' The issue is not that the man is free to do anything he feels like. It all depends on your motive.[65]

Knowing that we are loved by God gives us the strength to live our own authentic lives without worrying what other people think. (And it allows us to give the same gift to others. We can never truly have dialogue with others if we are not secure in ourselves.) Once we have brought our shadow selves to God, and found that he loves us and wants us to *be* us, then we don't have to worry about our real selves being somehow exposed. We've already been there, done that, bought the hair shirt. We have faced the darkness and come out the other side.

But freedom is not licence. God's love cannot be an

excuse for selfishness. The key here is following Jesus. Our freedom to act extends only so far as we are actually living the life of Christ. Which, as I hope to show in the next chapter, goes quite a long way. Augustine's saying 'Love – and do what you will' only works if we get the 'love' bit right. We want to *selve*, not be selfish. We are freed from the pressures of conformity so that we can call people to the rebel Jesus.

Like all things, the freedom to live an authentic life can have its shadow side. Suicide bombers believe that God loves them and approves of what they are doing, even though a few moments' thought ought to show them how tragically stupid that view is. You cannot earn God's approval by becoming the devil incarnate. That applies to those poor, defrauded, deluded adolescents who strap on the Semtex and walk to the checkpoint. Equally, those who believe that God loves them so much they can do exactly what they want are missing the point. Frankly, this applies to any of us who think that freedom gives us licence to pursue our dreams by wrecking the lives of others.

So. Listen to God. Follow Jesus' example. Be attentive to the most important people in your life. Be open to correction and ready to learn. Do the best work you can do. But for heaven's sake (literally), stop worrying about what other people think of you. This is not the same as doing what you like, or 'not giving a damn'. It is, rather, the freedom to be more yourself and more like Jesus each day. Don't worry about what people think of you, worry about what they think of Jesus when they meet you.

For me, I have finally stopped worrying about what people think of me. Almost. A bit. I want to be the best

Nick I can be. I want to write the best, most helpful, most truthful words I can. I want to be more like Jesus. And I want to build a really good shed.

One of the characteristic feelings of middle age is a desire for a bit of adventure, a willingness to step out in a new direction. We have that now: the challenge is to be truly ourselves and truly Jesus. So now I want to look at *how* we take hold of this new life that lies before us. Earlier we looked at the MAMILs (middle-aged men in lycra), out on the road urging themselves to greater physical achievements. Terrific. In the next section we'll look at a different set of exercises, ones which will help us to be more like Christ. Which is body-building of an entirely different sort.

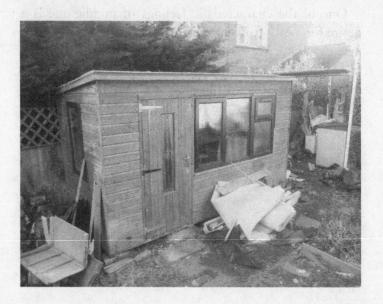

7

DANCING

The desert

This morning it is frosty outside. The sky is a brilliant, almost Mediterranean blue. The frost draws intriguing patterns on the debris that covers the garden so it's like a building site. There is a beauty among the bits of old carpet and offcuts of plywood and the shattered remains of old pallets.

The grass under my feet is brittle, crystallised, sugared with ice. It crunches beneath me. I sip my coffee and let my breath fog the air. Inside the shed I sit down and try to centre myself. The candle burns slowly, steadily. It feels like I have entered a plunge pool, a spiritual ice bath after a sauna. The words of Psalm 131 fight against all the other distractions of my mind.

'Lord, my heart is not lifted up, my eyes are not raised . . .'

My feet are cold.

'. . . too high. I do not occupy myself with things . . .'

Something scutters across the roof. Two blackbirds suddenly spin down past the window.

'. . . too great and too marvellous . . .'

My back aches. I shift in my seat. Sit still.

'. . . for me. But I have calmed and quieted my soul, like a . . .'

My feet are really cold. Sit still.

'. . . weaned child with its mother; my soul is like the weaned child that is with me . . .'

I may have frostbite. I will die here in the cold. In years to come they will find my remains perfectly preserved, like that bog man discovered in the Alps, shrink-wrapped in his blackened skin . . .

'O Israel, hope in the LORD . . .'

SIT STILL . . .

'. . . from this time on and for evermore.'

Hard work. I'm not very good at it, but even so, the shed has become my cell, my place of change. It is my desert in the back garden. But it's hard to stay focused.

After a while I think about work. The birds are singing in the garden. One of the joys of spending time in the shed is the nearness of birdsong. Blackbirds, chaffinches, the short morse-code *tseep* of the blue tit, further away a great tit sounding like someone pumping up an airbed. At one point a shadow passes over the garden: a red kite, gliding, flapping its wings in a desultory manner. In the early morning sun its rust-coloured wings are stretched out, fingertips reading the air currents like Braille. There is such beauty in the world.

And pain too. On the end wall of the shed is a cross. I made it quickly, out of the roughest, most basic wood I could find. A piece of two-by-one battening, scarred and splintered, pockmarked rusty brown with the stains where the nails had been during its previous life. The mortice joint is rough and haphazard.

I made it like this because this was how it would have been done at the time. Wood was scarce in Palestine in Jesus' day. You recycled it. The crossbeam that Jesus carried to the place of his execution – carried some of the way, before Simeon from Cyrenia was plucked from the crowd to do the job – would have been used on previous victims. Its nail holes would have been stained a dark, brownish red.

No one can follow me unless they take up their cross . . .

It reminds me of why I am here. I am here to learn how to be like this man. I am here to join the dance of the world in both its beauty and its pain. I am a writer, shed-builder, dancer. Disciple.

A change of career

Some time ago I went to a micro-brewery on the outskirts of Oxford to pick up a polypin of beer for a party.* The brewery was in a small converted barn, not much bigger than a double garage. The room held two huge, gleaming stainless-steel vats and the air was perfumed with hops. I got chatting to the owner, who was probably called Steve, as he packaged my order.

'Have you always worked for a brewery?'

'No,' he replied. 'I used to be a management consultant.'

---

* There are 8 pints in a gallon. A polypin is 4.5 gallons, or about 20 litres. Just enough to whet the appetite, really. In beer measurement, a polypin is half a firkin, which is a quarter of a barrel. There: inspirational *and* educational.

'Right. Bit of a career change, then.'

'Yes,' he smiled. 'I got really tired of telling people stuff they already knew. And I was even more tired of driving up and down the M4.'

I could see his point: the commute, the sense of aimlessness, a job which was no longer fulfilling. For a fleeting moment I entertained dreams of starting my own brewery. But I am better at drinking beer than making it. Stick to your gifts, that's my motto. Still, if you're going to have a mid-life career change, brewing seems a fine choice.

One of the most characteristic indicators of advancing mid-lifiness is a desire for change. Sometimes pursuing this can really help, because the change of pace, the sense of being your own boss, the joy of doing something you really care about – that's got to be a good thing. But it also brings other stresses. Being your own boss is one thing, but that means shouldering all the burdens. I've met plenty of people who have given up their life in the city to follow their dream. And I've met quite a few people who have returned when their dream turned out to be, if not a nightmare, then less dreamy than they imagined. We love the idea of chucking in the job, moving to the country and pursuing our dream of making Raku pottery, but the Inland Revenue will still come calling, the bills need to be met. There is always a price to pay for dreams.

More importantly, a career change, in and of itself, is not likely to solve all your problems. And what if you actually like your job? Changing career is no good if the problem is you. Let's ponder another Arnold Schwarzenegger film. In *Total Recall*, he goes to a company which promises you the ultimate holiday. 'What is it that is exactly the same about every single vacation you have ever taken?' asks the salesman. 'You! You're the same. No matter where you go, there you are. It's always the same old you.' Wherever we go, there we are. Change your job, change your wife, travel to Mars in a 1990s movie, move to the country and take up beekeeping – your shadow side will always go with you. The solution, then, is not to change our circumstances, but to deal with ourselves. But how do we do that?

The change we need to pursue lies not in our career, but in ourselves. Jesus calls us into the most significant personal professional development of our life. Forget Sir Alan, Jesus calls us to be his apprentice. Or, as he called it, a disciple.

In the Gospels, Jesus meets someone who is stuck in a dead-end job in every sense. Levi, son of Alphaeus, is sitting at his tollbooth one day when Jesus passes by. In the world of first-century Judaism, tax collectors were outcasts. Reviled for their dishonesty and widely shunned by other Jews, they were viewed as ritually impure. In the *Mishnah* – the collection of rabbinical law – it says, 'If a tax-gatherer enter a house, [all that is within] the house becomes unclean.' The reason was simple: tax collectors were cheats and frauds. Worst of all, they were working, ultimately, for the occupying Roman forces. Levi was pretty low down in the food chain of this world, too. His job was to collect the duties owed on goods travelling across the territorial borders – in this case, the border between the territory ruled by Herod Philip and that ruled by Herod Antipas. Like border guards and customs officers in many parts of the world today, it was a job with ample opportunity to take bribes and kick-backs.

What must Levi's life have been like? He had friends, probably, mainly in his own profession – after all, who else would have anything to do with him? Even those orthodox Jews who did not despise him would still have avoided his company because of his impurity. Levi's story is that he is hated. And people who are hated learn mainly how to hate.

And then one day Jesus walks by. And he says two words to Levi: 'Follow me.' That's all. No promises of reward or threats of retribution. No lectures on morality or patriotic duty. Nothing except 'Follow me'.

So he did. He rose from his booth and followed Jesus. What was he thinking? He had a safe career, after all. As Benjamin Franklin was to say a long time later, the only two certainties in life are death and taxes. But Levi was no longer interested in certainty. When a man who did not despise him walked into his life, Levi was ready for risk.

Levi followed Jesus and the path led – well, it led to Levi's house, actually, where Levi hosted a dinner for Jesus. In direct contravention of the purity laws, Jesus was prepared to eat with Levi and with other 'tax collectors and sinners' (Mark 2:15). He reclined with them, he was not distant or aloof. No wonder the scribes were outraged. Jesus replied, 'Those who are well have no need of a physician, but those who are sick; I have come to call not the righteous but sinners' (Mark 2:17).

There you go. That's why Levi followed Jesus. Because Jesus called him into a different story, a story where Levi could be healed of his loneliness and pain. Levi's calling to adventure was to become a disciple.

I have read a lot of discipleship books. A *lot*. And hardly any of them actually explain what Jesus meant by the word 'disciple'. The Greek word is *mathētēs*. At its root is the word *manthano* – 'to learn'. But it implies more than just a theoretical, ooh-that's-quite-interesting kind of learning. It indicates a significant, personal, whole-life commitment. Herodotus, in whose writings the term first appears, uses the word to describe Anacharsis, a barbarian nomadic Scythian raider, who went to Greece on a holiday – or possibly a savage raiding party – and fell head over heels in love with Greek culture. He became 'a *mathētēs* of the ways of Greece', so taken by the civilisation that he moved there.[66] He loved the product so much he bought the company.

Very early in its history the noun *mathētēs* was commonly used to indicate a person who was a learner or apprentice. In those times, apprentices learnt by imitation. The goal was to turn yourself into a close replica of your teacher. This was particularly true of the disciples who gathered around the famous rabbis of Jesus' day. A famous sage would allow several chosen followers to live in, or near, his house, and to follow him around all day while they discussed any questions of law together. The disciples' aim was not just to listen to their rabbi's words and join in the debates, but to imitate their master's behaviour and way of life. Sometimes it was less like learning and more like stalking. One disciple followed his master into the toilet; another hid under his rabbi's marital bed. When the rabbi and, presumably, his wife, objected, the disciple justified his actions by saying, 'But this is Torah, and I must learn!'

The same approach lies behind Jesus' idea of discipleship. For Jesus, the role of a disciple was to follow him and do the things he did. 'A disciple is not above the teacher,' he said, 'but everyone who is fully qualified will be like the teacher' (Luke 6:40). A disciple is involved in a natural process that will bring him or her to be like the master.

And they, in turn, are to pass it on. Jesus told his followers to 'Go and make disciples' and they knew only one way of doing that: observation and imitation. So, when Paul writes, 'Be imitators of me, as I am of Christ' (1 Corinthians 11:1), he is not being big-headed, he is merely reflecting how discipleship works. Other early church writers used the same terminology. Ignatius of Antioch urged believers to be 'imitators of the Lord', while a book called *The Martyrdom of Polycarp* describes martyrs as 'disciples and imitators of the Lord'.[67] Disciples are linked into a chain of imitative behaviour.

All of which means that Jesus' command to 'Go and make disciples' does *not* mean 'Go and tell people more and more facts about me', or 'Go and get people to agree with a load of statements about me'.

It means, 'Go and show people what it is to be like me. Go and make apprentices.' To be a disciple is to be a trainee Jesus. An apprentice Christ.

And we do not learn alone. In Jesus' day, disciples learnt with others, working out their apprenticeship as part of a learning community. Jesus has a school of disciples. Only he calls his school a kingdom.

The kingdom of God

The concept of the kingdom of God is crucial to the teaching of Jesus. Indeed, the first time he let his disciples off the leash to go and try some fieldwork, the message was, 'Go and tell people that the kingdom of God is near.'

The kingdom was near, but also already present. 'If it is by the finger of God that I cast out the demons, then the kingdom of God has come to you,' said Jesus, immediately after casting a demon out of someone (Luke 11:20). The kingdom is for now, and for the future, and for all stops in between. It has arrived in part, but is also still arriving. One day it will be fully realised, but at the moment the cosmos, like its inhabitants, is still working towards its individuation.

So if the kingdom is here now, then where is it? If we look for it in institutions we will be disappointed. We should not confuse the kingdom of God with the organised church of whatever flavour, and certainly not with the church building down the street. It can exist and flourish in these places, of course, but history shows us that the church can also be a very ungodly place indeed. The kingdom is not a building, not an institution, not a denomination, not even anyone who simply labels themselves 'Christian'. That's not the kingdom of God. How could it be? If the kingdom of God included anyone who labelled themselves as Christian, then it would have to include the 'Protestants' and 'Catholics' in Ireland who went around kneecapping each other, or the Lord's

Resistance Army in Uganda, who abduct children and brutalise them into becoming soldiers, or the American televangelist who promises some poor sucker in a trailer park that the Lord will bless them if only they send their $10.

Nor, I think, is the kingdom some invisible, other-wordly parallel dimension. (The Bible does have a word for that, and that word is 'heaven'. Heaven, rightly understood, is not 'up there' but alongside this earth.) The kingdom is very much *not* an abstract, spiritual realm, like Nirvana or the seventh heaven or some transcendental state of I'm-all-rightness. I mean, God might take you into those states, but that's not where Jesus says the kingdom of God is to be found. Nor is it to be found in doctrinal purity and behaving religiously. You can know all there is to know about theology, you can master all the -isms and rise to the highest ranks of the clergy and still behave in an ungodly way. The kingdom of God is not limited to the space between our ears.

No, the kingdom of God is not buildings, but behaviour. Remember the scribe whom Jesus said was 'not far from the kingdom of God'? He was nearly but not quite across the border. He had given the right answer, discovered the right information, but now he had to act on it.

The kingdom of God comes into existence where people are trying to be like Jesus. The prayer that Jesus taught his followers is a prayer of commitment to kingdom behaviour: 'Your kingdom come. Your will be done on earth, as it is in heaven' (Matthew 6:10). The kingdom is seen on earth where God's will is done. And that means it is enacted in this world, made visible, only in the lives of the citizens. As Dallas Willard writes, 'Our "kingdom" is simply the range of our effective will. Whatever we genuinely have the say over is in our kingdom.'[68] The kingdom of God is encountered in the Jesus-shaped lives of its citizens.

For Jesus, people entered the kingdom when they submitted their lives to the rule of God. 'He has rescued us from the power of darkness and transferred us into the kingdom of his beloved Son,' writes Paul (Colossians 1:13), while 1 Peter states that 'you are a chosen race, a royal priesthood, a holy nation, God's own people' (1 Peter 2:9).

But we have to choose to live in this kingdom. Jesus calls you, but you need to respond. The choice to follow Jesus, to be a disciple, is the single most authentic, most important, most *individuating* act you can ever make. No one can make that decision for you. Even God cannot make it for you – or will not. We *choose* to follow Jesus. It is an act of will. Many people find themselves going to church. Some people just sort of end up 'believing' in Jesus. But nobody drifts into discipleship. It's a crisis. A *krinein*. A decision point.

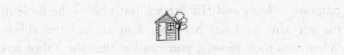

Jesus and his friends

Does the word 'disciple' sound off-putting? Well, it's a way of expressing a relationship between a master and a trainee, and no one, I think, would argue that we have nothing to learn from Jesus of Nazareth. But if you think it's a bit formal, the good thing is that Jesus himself didn't leave it at that. In John's Gospel, in a long speech that Jesus gave on the night before his execution, he said this:

> No one has greater love than this, to lay down one's life for one's friends. You are my friends if you do what I command you. I do not call you servants any longer, because the servant does not know what the master is doing; but I have called you friends, because I have made known to you everything that I have heard from my Father. (John 15:13-15)

We are disciples, yet more than disciples. We are Jesus' friends. Nothing, for me, sums this up better than a fifth-century Coptic icon which is to be found in the Louvre, Paris. The icon shows Jesus and the leader of a monastery – Abba Menas. In the Louvre, the title of the painting is *Jesus and His Friend*. Jesus holds the Bible in his left arm, and has his right arm around the abbot. When you look closely, you can see that the abbot has something peculiar about his eyes: one eye looks out at the world, the other eye looks sideways towards Jesus. It's not that the abbot had eye problems, it's symbolic: all of

Jesus' apprentices have one eye on the world and one eye on their master.

Normally, in an icon, Jesus' right hand would be raised in the sign of blessing. But here, he cannot do that: his right arm is flung around the abbot's shoulders. So here, it is the abbot who gives the traditional sign of blessing. We pass on Christ's blessing to the world. His arm around our shoulders gives us the reassurance, the strength, the confidence to pass on his love to those we meet.

So, if we are going to be apprentices of Jesus, what tasks do we have to do? What actions should we imitate? How do we deepen our friendship with Jesus? How do we begin to become the person God wants us to be? In other words, 'What next?'

Well, we have done the wrestling. We have embraced the embracing. It is time, my friends, to dance.

Learning to dance

While I was working on the shed, The Wife and I had our thirtieth wedding anniversary. The Wife likes to see me gainfully employed, so among her gifts to me was an index card box, and in it, alphabetically arranged, a list of activities to be done on our 'Date Nights' through the year. One of those was 'Learn Modern Jive'. So off we went to a class.

Now, my teenage years were in the 1970s, when the

standard approach at school discos was to lean against the wall and watch the girls dance around their handbags until it got to the end of the evening, when the DJ put on a slow track and there was a mad, feral rush for the particular girl you fancied. Then you held each other close(ish), and waddled around in a small circle. That was my only real experience of dancing 'in hold', not to say holding on for dear life. Later, attending gigs in grubby concert halls, I learnt to pogo while punk bands tried to make my ears bleed.

Neither experience really prepared me for Modern Jive. This kind of dancing is a lot more demanding. There are many interestingly named moves to master: Octopus, Hatchback, Yo-yo, Catapult. And you learn, of course, by copying. You watch the instructors on the stage and you then imitate their moves. Some of us are better at it than others. You will not be surprised to hear that my movements are A Thing Of Wonder. On our first lesson, as I moved around the floor, there were audible gasps of admiration at how far I had come in just two hours. Several people sensed a disturbance in the Force. A new Dance Messiah had come among them. It was like *The Matrix*, with twirls – I was kind of a dancing Neo.

Or not. It was flipping hard work. I wasn't bad, actually, but it is very demanding. At first you feel self-conscious and unnatural and unco-ordinated, and it seems like all you are doing is counting and concentrating and then getting it wrong. But there are odd moments when you do actually move in a co-ordinated way, when you respond to each other, when you stop thinking about it and just do it. When you are actually dancing.

In this final section of the book I want to take a very brief look at some of the ways in which we can experience God's presence, deepen our friendship with Jesus and enter more fully into the kingdom of God. Typically, these practices are called the spiritual disciplines – a name which makes them sound about as appealing as a bowl of cold porridge. Actually, they are the stuff we do to take hold of the love of God and to let his life flow through us.

These are the basic dance moves of the kingdom of God.

OK. I can sense, already, a renewed anxiety among my male readers. *He mentioned dancing*. It's all right, it's OK, take some deep breaths, calm down. It's just a metaphor. You are not being asked to dance. There. Better?

If this idea makes you come over all British and uncomfortable, then maybe concentrate on the apprenticeship side. The thing is, being a disciple of Jesus does have an element of work about it. There is stuff you are supposed to do. What I'm trying to get across through the idea of the dance thing is that the more you do this stuff, the more natural, and even joyous, it becomes.

God does not want robots. He wants dancers. That means we're allowed to get things wrong. We are clumsy – particularly at first – with two left feet and no sense of rhythm. But gradually we learn not to worry too much about that.

So here we go. Here is some stuff for you to try out. I'm going to suggest seven areas and some simple exercises to get you started. The seven areas I'm going to focus on are:

Sitting: solitude and silence
Listening: prayer and contemplation
Reading: encountering God in the Bible
Serving: work and the daily grind
Self-control: simplicity and generosity
Making: creativity and craftsmanship
Celebrating: joy and thanksgiving

You might find some of these exercises hard. You might experience some discomfort, either physical or psychological. Maybe both at once. That's OK. Stay with it. Or you might be very experienced in this kind of spiritual formation stuff. In which case, feel free to invent your own moves. We don't have to get prescriptive about this; within each area I'm sure you will find your own path. Here's a lesson from the Desert Fathers:

> Nesteros, the friend of the renowned Antony of Egypt, was asked what work monks should do. He replied, 'Surely all works please God equally? Scripture says, Abraham was hospitable and God was with him; Elijah loved quiet and God was with him; David was humble and God was with him.' So whatever you find you are drawn to in God's will, do it and let your heart be at peace.[69]

Exercise #1. Sitting: solitude and silence

Jesus was baptised by John. It was a significant moment: the Holy Spirit descended on him, the voice of God spoke out. You'd have expected Jesus to leap out of the water and go, 'Right. You heard what the big guy said. Let's get cracking.'

Instead he went into the wilderness and spent forty days on his own. Throughout his life, according to the Gospels, Jesus withdrew to quiet places. He went there at crisis points. After the death of his friend and cousin John the Baptist, before choosing his twelve core disciples, when the crowds exhausted him or tried to force him to be king, in the weeks before the climactic journey to Jerusalem, on the night before his execution – these were all occasions when Jesus withdrew to a place of stillness and quiet.

Solitude and silence are absolutely crucial for surviving and thriving in the second half of life. We have looked at our need to reflect on the deep questions of identity and anxiety – 'Who are you?', 'What are you afraid of?' It is in solitude and silence that we come before God to find the answers. It is in the 'recreating stillness of solitude', to use Richard Foster's powerful phrase, that God remakes us, renames us.[70]

We are not used to this. Our lives are characterised by noise and activity. Every day we are assaulted by information. Emails bombard us. The phone screams like a crying child. Back at home, we switch the TV on, or the radio. Maybe we nervously check Facebook or Twitter every five minutes, in case we are missing out on something. We're always plugged in, connected.

Am I missing something good? Have I gained any new followers? Have I been noticed? *Do I really matter?*

The core activity of the Desert Fathers was solitude.

> A brother went to [Abba] Moses to ask for his advice. He said to him, 'Go and sit in your cell and your cell will teach you everything.'[71]

Turn it off. Turn it all off. Go off the grid. Unplug yourself.

Solitude, proactively and deliberately chosen, is, if you like, the flip side of the dark night. In the dark night our solitude cages us, scares us, crushes us. But when we seek solitude ourselves, then it liberates, encourages, empowers. As Henri Nouwen said, 'Solitude is . . . the place of purification and transformation, the place of the great struggle and the great encounter.'[72]

At first you might find this disorientating, even scary. We are so addicted to sound, sights and sensation, that coming off it cold turkey is very difficult. But gradually you get accustomed to it. Distractions will still be there, but they will dissipate more quickly. The solitude expands, opens up before you, allowing space in which to bring before God all the deepest issues of life.

As you become more experienced at it you will find that there are little moments of solitude in the day when you can just drink a refreshing draught of quietness. Walking can offer what the philosopher Frédéric Gros calls a 'suspensive freedom' – allowing you to escape the information overload, and providing a place where you can be a constructive 'nobody'.[73] But equally, walking is active and stimulating, and part of what we need is stillness.

The intentional times of concentrated solitude are important. You might even want to extend the period of time you spend alone. Many people find it helpful to go on a silent retreat, spending a weekend or a couple of days in silence at a monastery or retreat centre.

THE INSTRUCTIONS

Here's what we're going to do. Every day, for a week, we're going to go somewhere quiet and sit in absolute silence for ten minutes.

- Find a time and a place where you won't be disturbed. (I don't know if I've mentioned this, but I have a shed . . .)
- Don't take your phone. Don't take anything with you.
- Sit on a chair in a relaxed, but not too relaxed, posture.
- Close your eyes and just concentrate on your breathing. If it helps, focus on a key word, like 'peace', or think about God by saying his name or the name of Jesus. Some people use a very short repeated prayer.
- After a few seconds, I guarantee that your mind will start to drift. You will suddenly notice all the noise in your head, all the things you have to do, the thoughts you carry around with you. This is absolutely natural, but don't dwell on them: try to just let these go.

- Similarly, you might notice noise elsewhere: birdsong, traffic noise, distant voices. Let that be as well.
- Carry on focusing on your breathing. Slow it down. And just sit still.
- Do that for ten minutes every day. You might find it helpful to set a timer to tell you when ten minutes is up.

Solitude is not a complete withdrawal. Personally I never have a problem with my own company. Most writers are happy on their own, it sort of goes with the territory. If anything I go the other way, not wanting to see people or do things. But we go into silence and solitude in order to nourish our interaction with others, not to run away from them.

Solitude is best when it is rooted in community. John Burnside wrote of a friend in the Arctic who said, 'Here, it's not about solitude, its about having a real community. Once you have a community, *then* you can be alone . . . When you go out to the edge of the world, you have to have something to come back to. You may not come back very often, but you have to know that you can. Otherwise, you're lost.'[74]

We do not want to be lost. We want to be found.

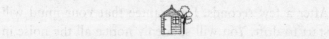

Exercise #2. Listening: prayer and contemplation

'Ask, and it will be given you,' said Jesus, 'search, and you will find; knock, and the door will be opened for you. For everyone who asks receives, and everyone who searches finds, and for everyone who knocks, the door will be opened' (Matthew 7:7-8).

Jesus' habit was to pray, and pray frequently. 'In the morning, while it was still very dark, he got up and went out to a deserted place, and there he prayed,' says Mark's Gospel (1:35). If we look at the great saints and heroes of Christianity, the one thing they all have in common is a reliance on prayer.

Some people get really excited about prayer. I have to admit, I am not, usually, among their number. There's a very simple test to find out if you are a prayer warrior or not. Just answer this question honestly: prayer or pub? Yep. Me too. (Of course, it's a false distinction. It's perfectly possible, in fact, to go to the pub and pray.)

I think part of the problem is that no one teaches us how to pray. Jesus' disciples asked him to teach them a prayer – and he gave them what we now call the Lord's Prayer. That's a great start for when you don't know how to pray. But prayer, in general, is something that must be learnt. And like everything worth doing in life – cricket, dancing, shed building – you only get better at it by doing it.

Another reason we don't engage in prayer is because we don't understand it. Prayer is a mystery. The Bible urges us to pray – and people in need naturally do – but no one has ever understood why sometimes it works and sometimes it doesn't. For men, this can be a problem, because we are people who expect to fix things. That's what we do. Indeed, our religious culture often promotes a view of prayer which is primarily about fixing things or asking for stuff. And when we don't get the answers we need, when prayer *doesn't* seem to fix things, that's a problem. But I have come to realise that prayer is not, primarily, about fixing, asking or even getting answers. It's about meeting God.

In the Bible, Job and his 'companions' spend thirty-seven chapters arguing about why so many disasters have been visited on him. They want God to justify himself, to explain why a good man has been treated so shabbily. Finally, in chapter 38, God does make an appearance. He appears 'out of the whirlwind'. Far from answering anyone's questions, God accuses them all of talking rubbish and then says, 'Gird up your loins like a man, I will question you, and you shall declare to me' (Job 38:3). In other words, prepare to wrestle. And Job is fine with this.

Job comes to understand that the presence of God drives out all the questions. It's not that the questions don't matter, and it's certainly not the case that Job was wrong to be asking them. Rather, it's that there is something deeper than that, a base layer of life on which and at which the questions rest.

That base layer is the relationship between us and God. True, deep prayer occurs when there is just us and God, when, instead of offering ourselves to the world for its judgement, we offer ourselves to God.

THE INSTRUCTIONS

There are loads of ways to pray. I'm going to suggest that you explore the daily prayer of self-examination.* It is a simple set of steps to help you review the day.

At the end of the day, find a quiet place to reflect.

- Look back at the day that is past. Try and recall what happened. Don't *judge* at this stage, just recall the events.
- Give thanks for the day. Be grateful.
- Drill down a bit. Have a closer examination of the day. What did you do? What was done to you? How did you react?
- Own up. Could you have done things differently? Did you behave at your best? Did you fail? Face up to what is wrong.
- Finally, let it go. That's gone now. Time to look forward. Based on what you now know about yourself, ask God to be with you in the day to come.

---

* The posh name for this is The Prayer of Examen. Not so much a title, more a spelling mistake. It comes from Ignatius, although *examen* is a Latin word meaning 'balance', so I don't know why we don't just translate it. In fact, earlier translations of Ignatius seem not to have used the word. The earliest records of the word in English come from 1651 and 1669 and refer to Saint Teresa and someone called Father Paul. According to the *Oxford English Dictionary*, the first mention of it in relation to Ignatius comes from 1885. Anyway, we're not at home to Mr Pretentious.

Prayer is about honesty. In that crucial wrestling match Jacob has the temerity to demand things of God, and then the courage to admit who he is before God. 'Jacob shows us how to pray,' writes John Sanford. 'If we are angry with God, say so; if we love him, say so; if we are afraid, bring this into our prayer. Prayer is relationship with God and no relationship, certainly not with the Divine, exists without emotional honesty.'[75]

Exercise #3. Reading: encountering God in the Bible

Another core practice of Jesus: reading the Scriptures. Jesus quoted the Scriptures a lot.* He had clearly studied them and memorised them. And he used them in his prayers. He carried them within him.

He rejected temptation in the wilderness with quotes from Deuteronomy and from the Psalms. He used Scriptures to correct people, to challenge them and to give them insight. He even acted out Scriptures: when riding into Jerusalem he chose to act out a passage predicting the Messiah from the book of Zechariah. He used them for consolation; on the cross, he cried out a passage from a Psalm.

The great theologian Karl Barth once attempted to

---

* Of course, in his day, he was using the Jewish Scriptures – the Tanakh, what we call the Old Testament.

describe what was different about the Bible: 'What is there within the Bible?' he asked. 'What sort of house is it to which the Bible is the door? What sort of country is spread before our eyes when we throw the Bible open?' [76] Good question, Karl.

Barth called his essay 'The Strange New World within the Bible', which is a very good description of this book. The Bible is like a foreign country. And that can cause us problems, because sometimes middle-aged men and foreign countries do not go together too well. We don't speak the language, we can't find our way around, the food tastes funny, the locals are weird and the plumbing doesn't work. We don't mind certain places, but we stay in the most popular bits – the beaches or the bars – and we don't venture off the beaten track.

Well, let's push that idea for a moment. When we go to explore a foreign country, we will get much more out of it if we go prepared. Yes, we can just drop in, hit the tourist spots, get a quick blessing from the gift shop and go home. We'll get something out of that. But we'll gain much, much more if we go to the land – the strange land of the Bible – and *live* there.

Just as with prayer, we have not been taught properly how to read the Scriptures. We tend to think of the Bible as a great big book of doctrine, or a compendium of theology, or God's Enormous Book of Answers. But the Bible is a meeting place. The main reason, for Christians, why we read the Bible is because we believe that God speaks to us through this book.

There is a story told in East Africa about a woman who always used to walk around the village with her Bible. She carried it everywhere. 'Why are you always reading that?' her neighbours teased her. 'There are so many other books you could read.' The woman replied, 'I know there are many books I could read. But this is the only book which reads me.'

Daily Bible reading is a really good habit to get into. But simply reading the Bible is never going to change your life. That only happens when you *listen* to what God is saying through it. So we're going to learn some Bible verses, carry them with us and listen for how God speaks through them.

THE INSTRUCTIONS

- Choose a Bible passage. Here are some good ones for this exercise: John 3:16; John 10:10; Philippians 4; Psalm 131. But you can choose any you want.
- Read the passage.
- Now read it again, slowly. Pause as you go along. Try to learn it.
- Get a piece of paper or card and copy it out. Carry that card with you, or put it somewhere around the house.
- As time permits, keep trying to remember it through the day. Just 'listen' to it in your head and see if God speaks to you through it.
- Rinse and repeat!

In medieval monasteries, the process of meditating on Scriptures was known as 'rumination'. Monks would repeat the Scripture to themselves over and over again. This has been described as 'a slow and noisy process – an audible "chewing over" of the precious words of the text'.

One monk wrote that the Bible should be 'in your heart by memory, in your mouth by devout rumination, and in your deeds by affectionate imitation'.[77]

As all men know, it helps if you have the right tool for the job. So get hold of a good translation – there are loads available. You do not have to read the King James Version. The Bible was not written in an archaic language and you don't have to read it that way either.* And don't worry about the bits that you can't understand. The truth is, there are some bits that *no one* really understands. This is a very ancient text. But for me it's not the bits of the Bible that I don't understand that cause me concern: it's the bits I understand very well, but don't do!

Exercise #4. Serving: work and the daily grind

Jesus worked for a living. He spent some fifteen years of his life as a builder in the Nazareth-based firm Joseph and Sons. This was not some unimportant interlude between his birth and his later public mission: it was a crucial time, in which he was a normal part of his society. It is very likely that Jesus and his father worked on the building sites of Sepphoris, a major city near Nazareth, when it was being rebuilt. Images from the building world

---

* The New Testament was actually written in a language called *koiné* Greek – an everyday dialect used by the traders and merchants and common folk around the Mediterranean world.

nourish his sayings and his stories: he talked about what happens to houses with inadequate foundations, how you should estimate the cost before you begin building, how you can't remove the sawdust speck from your brother's eye when you have a whacking great beam of wood in your own.*

Jesus seems to have given up his work as a builder for the final three years of his life. But then, on the night before his death, he took on a quite different role. A shocking role. He took off his outer clothing and washed the feet of his disciples. In the society of the time, no free man would ever wash the feet of others. The only men who would do that were slaves. Jesus deliberately adopts the posture of a worker on the lowest rung of the empire.

Our workplaces are furnaces of spiritual transformation. Work is where we learn so many things: patience, humility, service.

I am very good at serving others, just as long as people see me doing it. I can do humility, as long as I get praise. But the seventeenth-century writer Jeremy Taylor said, 'Love to be concealed and little esteemed, be content to want [i.e. go without] praise, never be troubled when thou art slighted or undervalued . . .' Thanks for that, Jezza.

Our workplaces give us the opportunity to do just that: to serve others. So look for opportunities to serve others at work. Be attentive to the tasks you are given, and do them for the love of God. Even the harshest of conditions

---

* The word for 'beam' indicates the main crossbeam of the house: the ridge.

can be hallowed in this way. Paul wrote that slaves should 'obey your earthly masters in everything, not only while being watched and in order to please them, but whole-heartedly, fearing the Lord'. He told them that 'you serve the Lord Christ'.*

Even people called to a life of prayer have still worked. Monks talked of a life of two parts: *ora et labora* – 'work and prayer'. Perhaps the finest expression of this is the work of a Carmelite monk called Brother Lawrence. That was his monastic name. His real name was Nicholas. (I like him already.)

Nicholas Herman was born in 1611 in Lorraine, France. His family was poor and he had little education. He served in the French army but he was wounded in his thirties. Although he recovered, he was discharged from the army. He joined a monastery in Paris, where he spent most of the next forty years of his life as a washer-upper, cleaning the pots and the pans, sweeping the floor, serving in the kitchen. There he took on a new name – Brother Lawrence – and a new vocation: he was going to spend his life praying in the workplace.

After his death his colleagues published a volume of recollections of his conversations and letters. In this little book, *The Practice of the Presence of God*, we are invited to see a revolutionary view of work. Brother Lawrence set himself the task of communing with God wherever he was and whatever he was doing.

'The time of business does not with me differ from the

---

* But the same was true for masters: 'Masters, treat your slaves justly and fairly, for you know that you also have a Master in heaven' (Colossians 3:22 – 4:1).

time of prayer,' he wrote, 'and in the noise and clatter of my kitchen, while several persons are at the same time calling for different things, I possess God in as great tranquillity as if I were upon my knees at the blessed sacrament.'

THE INSTRUCTIONS

Let's go all 'Brother Lawrence', then. Here are a few things that you can do to practise the presence of God at your workplace.

- Like many men, I used to imagine myself as the next James Bond. Well, the good news is that our workplaces give us a real opportunity to join the secret service. Just not the MI6 variety. This week, do three acts of secret service in your workplace. Don't tell anyone. Take no credit.
- Do your tasks to the glory of God. Pray while you are in your meetings (probably not out loud; that can annoy the person chairing it).
- Try getting to a meeting a few minutes early and sit there. Not only do you go into the meeting itself more calm than others, but you get to feel incredibly smug.

While we're thinking of service, let's remember that our 'work' is not just what we do nine to five. There are other tasks which we can do to serve others: we can take on a cause, we can work for the poor, the homeless, those in need. It's good to get passionate about a cause. We're middle-aged men. We're grumpy anyway, we might as well be grumpy about something that matters.

The novelist Alice Walker joined a ship setting sail to

breach the Israeli blockade of Gaza. 'I am in my sixty-seventh year ...' she wrote. 'It seems to me that during this period of eldering it is good to reap the harvest of one's understanding of what is important, and to share this, especially with the young.'[78]

I love that word, *eldering*. It sounds rather Tolkienesque. One can imagine a group of men, dwarves, the occasional wizard, gathering for the eldering. And it sounds a damn sight better than 'getting old'. But she's not winding down. In other words, part of her eldering was to serve others and make a nuisance of herself in the cause of justice.

Exercise #5. Self-control: simplicity and generosity

Jesus spoke about money and possessions more than any other single issue. His words make for uncomfortable reading for the wealthy Western societies. The problem is not so much wealth in itself, but our slavish worship of it. 'No slave can serve two masters; for a slave will either hate the one and love the other, or be devoted to the one and despise the other. You cannot serve God and wealth' (Luke 16:13). For Jesus it was all about what demands our attention and our efforts. 'Where your treasure is, there your heart will be also,' he said (Matthew 6:21). Instead, we are urged to embrace radical generosity: 'Give to everyone who begs from you; and if anyone takes away your goods, do not ask for them again' (Luke 6:30).

He walked the talk. His was a life of simplicity. 'Foxes have holes, and birds of the air have nests; but the Son of Man has nowhere to lay his head' (Matthew 8:20). Which is not to say that Jesus had nothing. But what he had seems to have been given to him. Jesus knew how to give and how to receive. He was supported by the generosity of others. He was given clothes to wear. And in the end he even had to borrow a tomb. Just for a couple of days.

We crave a simpler, less demanding life. I read a book the other day about a man who spent five years living halfway up a Welsh mountain without running water, heating or electricity. I have since spent rather too much time on websites looking at derelict cottages out in the wilds ... The daydream of leaving it all behind and running off to live a life of freedom runs very deep! And it's ironic that achieving simplicity in our lives always seems to involve buying something new.

A team of anthropologists from the University of California, Los Angeles made a detailed survey of contemporary life and concluded that the society around them was 'the most materially rich society in global history, with light-years more possessions per average family than any preceding society'. I'm not sure quite how you measure possessions in light years, but then again, these people are in California, and that's the kind of thing they tend to say over there. Anyway, the smallest home in their study contained 2,260 items in its 980 square feet. And that was only the stuff they could see! They didn't count anything in drawers or cupboards. Nine out of ten of the families kept extra household items in the garage; three quarters of them had so much stuff that there was no room for the car.[79]

William Morris famously said, 'Have nothing in your house that you do not know to be useful or consider to be beautiful.' I've never applied this rule myself, on the grounds that I think I fail to qualify in both categories. But it is good to really *think* about what we own. Of course, just because we have few possessions doesn't automatically mean that we are living simply. A person can have hardly any actual possessions and still be living a life devoted to the love of money and anxious for its accumulation.

Simplicity is not just about physical space, but mental space as well. The apostle Paul identified this:

> Of course, there is great gain in godliness combined with contentment; for we brought nothing into the world, so that we can take nothing out of it; but if we have food and clothing, we will be content with these. But those who want to be rich fall into temptation and are trapped by many senseless and harmful desires that plunge people into ruin and destruction. For the love of money is a root of all kinds of evil, and in their eagerness to be rich some have wandered away from the faith and pierced themselves with many pains. (1 Timothy 6:6-10)

There are any number of books on decluttering. They hold out the promise of an organised life, where everything has its place and where we can always find our keys. And there are many ways in which we can simplify our lives. One of the simplest, appropriately enough, is to just give stuff away. Take a bag to the charity shop, give someone a surprise gift. Or operate a one-in, one-out policy: when you acquire a new item – a shirt, a book, a DVD – give another one away. (Or two . . .)

But unless we deal with the root problem, none of these off-the-peg solutions will work. It is good to declutter, but the question is, 'Why did I think it was a good thing to clutter in the first place?'

We fill our lives with stuff because we think that it is the way to cure our deep discontent. But the more stuff we have, the more complicated life becomes. Our lives are like a machine with too many moving parts: there is always something demanding maintenance. The Desert Father Evagrius suggests that desire is unsettling, noisy: 'Cut the desire for many things out of your heart and so prevent your mind being dispersed and your stillness lost.'[80] Simplicity allows us to concentrate on what is most necessary. Abba Poemen said, 'The beginning of all evil is to diversify the mind.'

The problem with this is that we can go too far the other way, and believe that there is something intrinsically good in poverty and asceticism. It is *not* good to be poor. It is soul-destroying, exhausting, demeaning and destructive. The call to simplicity is not about doing away with all this stuff, but about putting it in its rightful place. It's about *life*, because worshipping wealth and possessions will destroy us in the end. Simplicity is good because it brings freedom. It reorientates our lives towards what really matters.

'Simplicity is freedom,' advises Richard Foster. 'Duplicity is bondage. Simplicity brings joy and balance. Duplicity brings anxiety and fear.'[81]

Remember, life is more than our possessions. I like the story of Alexander the Great's visit to the philosopher Diogenes. Alexander had long wished to meet the famous philosopher, so when he visited Corinth he sought

Diogenes out. The great world-conqueror was a little surprised to discover that the renowned philosopher was little more than a beggar, a wizened man, brown as a nut, skin like leather, sitting under a tree dressed in nothing but rags. 'Can I do anything to help you?' asked Alexander.

'Yes,' replied Diogenes. 'Get out of the way, you're blocking the sun.'

THE INSTRUCTIONS

We're going to try fasting. This is simply abstaining from some form of consumption in order to focus on God. What you fast from is up to you – I'm going to suggest the traditional fasting from food, but you can fast from the internet, buying stuff, social media – whatever you feel you are over-consuming. I would suggest coffee, but that would be madness.

- Go without eating.* Drink water, but do not eat food.
- You can do this fast from lunch to lunch. Or refrain from food during the day, but eat a simple meal at night. This means you abstain from two meals.
- As you fast, monitor your inner response. How strong are the cravings? Use the time you would normally spend eating in prayer or study.

---

* It ought to go without saying that you should not do this if you are suffering from any health problems. Fasting is about self-control and self-denial, not self-abuse. The best advice on fasting is found in Richard Foster's book *Celebration of Discipline*.

Fasting not only addresses our need to consume, it builds in self-control. It teaches us how to say 'no'. Esau lost his birthright to Jacob because he had no self-discipline. 'I'm starving,' he wailed. Which was arrant nonsense.

Historically, fasting has always been part of discipleship. *The Didache*, an early Christian discipleship manual, recommends fasting on Wednesdays and Fridays.* The early church leader Polycarp urged Christians to be 'self-controlled in respect to prayer and persevere in fasting'. Another early church document, *The Shepherd of Hermas*, suggests that we should observe a 'partial fast' – eating just bread and water – and then estimate the money we would have spent on food and give it to the poor.[82]

A great way to bring together all the aspects of simplicity and self-control ...

Fasting is not dieting. We do not fast so that we can get into *Men and Fitness* magazine, nor do we simplify our house so that we can make the cover of *House Beautiful*. Through fasting we begin to learn how to do without everything except God. 'Fasting is one of the more important ways of practising that self-denial required of *everyone* who would follow Christ,' says Dallas Willard. 'In fasting we learn how to suffer happily as we feast on God.'[83] Jesus was very clear that we don't do it for show: 'When you fast, put oil on your head and wash your face, so that your fasting may be seen not by others but by your Father who is in secret; and your

---

* John Wesley felt so strongly about fasting that he refused to ordain anyone who did not follow the *Didache* and fast on those two days.

Father who sees in secret will reward you' (Matthew 6:17-18).

Fasting is an act of secret rebellion. It rebels against the idea that we need to keep consuming to be content and that the purpose of life is to satisfy ourselves.

Exercise #6. Making: creativity and craftsmanship

The creativity of Jesus is something that doesn't feature so much in the usual list of disciplines, yet it was one of his most characteristic activities. He was always making stuff. Sometimes he *literally* made things: his first miracle, according to John's Gospel, was to turn water into wine. More often, he fashioned beautifully crafted metaphors, stories that spoke directly into people's hearts, tales with such a creative power that even today, two millennia later, they can still amaze and inspire.

And Jesus had a history of craftsmanship. He worked, as we've seen, as a carpenter and builder. He must have learnt his trade, learnt how to use tools to make stuff. And, of course, if we go just a *tad* further back, we find the Bible presents Jesus as the Word, present with God at the moment of creation. So, *quite* creative, then.

God is Creator, and within us all, I believe, is a splinter of that creativity. We are created, the Bible says, in the image of God, and that must mean that we share his capacity for, and his love of, making.

Man is a maker. We love to build things: houses, gardens, stories, sheds. In a letter to artists written in 1999, Pope John Paul II wrote that, 'God ... called man into existence, committing to him the craftsman's task.'[84] There are surprisingly few books and little published thinking on the relationship between faith and creativity and craftsmanship, and what there is tends to be of the 'I'm An Artist Luvvie' mould. But I think creativity is more than wearing a smock and painting a picture of a daisy.

We are all called to be creative. At the most basic level we create the shape of our own life. As the Pope wrote, 'All men and women are entrusted with the task of crafting their own life: in a certain sense, they are to make of it a work of art, a masterpiece.' We all shape the 'wondrous material' of our own humanity.

Creativity is about the exercise of craftsmanship and skill. One of my favourite characters in the Bible is Bezalel, the man given the responsibility for designing and overseeing the production of all the stuff for the tabernacle. He is described as a man 'filled ... with divine spirit, with skill, intelligence, and knowledge in every kind of craft, to devise artistic designs, to work in gold, silver, and bronze, in cutting stones for setting, and in carving wood, in every kind of craft'. Bezalel had not only mastered these skills, he taught them to others as well (Exodus 35:30-35). In middle age we have an important role as mentors and teachers: we have learnt how to do things and we should be prepared to pass that knowledge on. We know how to problem-solve, and problem-solving is, essentially, a creative act.

Exercising our creativity gives us an important way in

which to express our deepest thoughts. Creativity helps us to see beauty. And men sometimes aren't very good at dealing with that. In his classic book, *God of Surprises*, Gerard Hughes tells of a taciturn Scotsman called Jock. At one point in their conversation, he opens up and relates how, after a relationship breakdown, he found himself 'walking the bloody moors wi' a wee dug'.* He came to the cliffs by the sea and had a deep feeling of wonder. 'The sea looked affie big and ah felt very wee but ah wis happy. Daft isn't it? Ah cannie tell my mates, cos they'd think ah wis kinky.'[85]

Here we have a man in touch with beauty, yet he cannot express that to others for fear of what they might think. I have to say, I've met a lot of middle-aged men like that. But our creative side can give us a language to use. Creativity connects us with beauty. We take a great photograph, paint a picture, write a poem. Or we watch the flowers that we planted come into bloom, we rejoice in a perfectly mitred joint or the way the grain runs through the wood as we plane it smooth. All of these are ways to honour and respect the creation around us.

Creativity is an expression of our own individuality. Through the exercise of our God-given creativity, we can do something unique, something only we could have come up with. Whether it's writing a song or making a chair or making a curry, if we allow the play of our imagination, we will find something nobody else can do.

Just don't use *too* much imagination with the curry.

* That's a dog. Not a tiny man called Douglas.

THE INSTRUCTIONS

I guess this is the one place where you shouldn't obey the instructions! Here are some ideas, but do what you want – express your creativity.

- Learn something new. Is there anything you want to try? Is there a skill or a craft you've always wanted to have a go at? Try it, or enrol on a course.
- Look for beauty. If there is a hobby that you already enjoy such as photography or writing or art, see how you can use that to see beauty. Take a photo which shows the beauty of the world, make a drawing which is uplifting and soul-enriching.
- Keep a journal. If you don't think you have a creative bone in your body, you might be surprised. Write what you did during your day and see how God spoke to you. Maybe even record your dreams. You may be surprised with what you discover.

The first thing God did was create. And that was more than an act of sheer invention and novelty. It brought order into the world, light into the darkness. To be creative is to see the wholeness and order of things, to give meaning to the world. But it's also to simply have fun. Middle-aged men *need* more fun in our lives. Allow yourself to be imaginative and playful. Watch *The LEGO Movie*, which is all about trashing the rulebook and using your imagination. Yes, watch *The LEGO Movie*: that's an order.

Exercise #7. Celebrating: joy and thanksgiving

Jesus' life was intimately linked with celebration. He observed the Jewish feasts. Each year he went up to Jerusalem to celebrate the festivals; each week it was his habit to observe Sabbath. According to John's Gospel, his first miracle was providing the wine for a wedding party; in Luke's Gospel he begins his public ministry by proclaiming the year of jubilee. Throughout, he talks about good news. 'The kingdom of heaven is like treasure hidden in a field, which someone found and hid; then in his joy he goes and sells all that he has and buys that field' (Matthew 13:44). The abundant life of Jesus is like a lottery win.

Before his death, he told his followers that what is coming will be like a joyous birth: 'When a woman is in labour, she has pain, because her hour has come. But when her child is born, she no longer remembers the anguish because of the joy of having brought a human being into the world. So you have pain now; but I will see you again, and your hearts will rejoice, and no one will take your joy from you' (John 16:20-22). Living in the power of the resurrected Christ is a perpetual birthday party.

'From its very beginning, Christianity has been the proclamation of joy, of the only possible joy on earth,' said Alexander Schmemann. The Easter liturgy of the Orthodox Church goes:

Enter ye all into the joy of your Lord,
You who are rich and you the poor, come to the feast,
Receive all the riches of loving-kindness ...
And let no one bewail his poverty,
For the universal Kingdom has been revealed.[86]

Brilliant. Triffic. Wonderful. So why are we so grumpy? Many middle-aged men are clinically grumpy. We can't help it. It's an instinctive, knee-jerk grumpiness. It starts because we don't like change, or we don't feel valued, or we don't feel involved, or we're just annoyed at the sheer, banal stupidity of modern life, but before we know it, grumpiness and cynicism are our default setting.

It doesn't have to be that way. Grumpiness is a choice. And Jesus calls us into joy.

I know, I know. Nothing is more irritating than being told to 'cheer up'. Like those posters that tell you to 'Think Positive'. You just want to take a flamethrower to them. But I want to let you into an important fact: it's true.

Positivity does change things. The brain has what is called 'neuroplasticity' – it continually adapts and evolves depending on our experiences, training and habits. In other words, repeated, habitual practices can modify the neuronal system of your brain and create new neural pathways.[87] To put it another way, we can actually change the way we think.

We have a choice of pathways available to us. We can continue to trudge down the well-worn path of negativity, but the more we choose that route, the more the positive path gets overgrown and harder to use. Instead, as Maureen Gaffney writes, 'By constantly building your capacity to experience positive emotion, you can clear and extend that lane way, see its beauty and pleasures and come to use it as your route of choice through life.'[88]

It takes some time, though, to change the muscle-memory of our own negativity. And we have to want to do it. Because we can get addicted to grumpiness. We get a kind of thrill about it. It makes us think that we know best, that we're not going to get taken in, unlike all those silly, hopelessly optimistic idiots.

Well, we're called to follow Jesus. To be like him. And whatever else he was, Jesus was not an old grumpy-pants who thought that everything was better in the olden days.

So let us seek to build positivity into our lives. There are many ways in which we can do this. We can spend more time with friends. We can practise optimism and choose to see the bright side first. We can change our attitudes and actually be nice to people. Our attitudes at work should speak to others of Jesus. We don't have to get sucked into the macho image of management that we see on *The Apprentice*. That's a gameshow, not real life.

Most of all, seek reasons to celebrate. When it comes to relationships it's very easy for couples to forget what it is that gave them joy in the first place. Make sure that you do stuff together. There are these things called babysitters. Book them. Get out for an evening, go away for a weekend.

One of the best celebrations is – or should be – Sabbath. In our money-rich, time-poor world, we have lost sight of Sabbath. We have already explored, a bit, how Jesus 'broke' the Sabbath, but he also held the Sabbath as well. The Sabbath is not only about rest, although, joyously, it certainly gives us that; it's a commemoration and celebration. In Jewish observance the Sabbath meal is a time to retell the story of their people and their relationship with God. It is a meal with a meaning. For Christians, the eucharist should be a celebratory experience. Despite the fact that it is often a sip of something that is not quite wine and a small piece of something that may once have been bread, it is meant to be a joyous reminder of death, resurrection and new life. It is a good idea to observe a proper Sabbath now and again. Start at sundown on the Saturday with a shared meal. Ignore the TV, spend time with each other. Drink wine. And give thanks.

THE INSTRUCTIONS

Build thankfulness into your life. Here are two ways to start opening up those overgrown neural pathways of joy.

- Say grace before your meals. *All* your meals – dinner, lunch, that coffee you just bought, that late-night bowl of cornflakes that you sneakily consumed. Because whether the food came from Sainsbury's, the Organic Artisanal Tofu Collective stall in the foodie market, or your own greenhouse, saying grace reminds us that what we have is a gift from God. He who keeps the earth spinning, the rain falling, the sun shining, the seasons . . . er . . . seasoning. Without this basic realisation we can never escape the addiction of accumulation.

- Begin and end each day by thanking God that you are alive. See if you can say 'thanks' the moment you open your eyes. And at the end of the day – and I know this is an old cliché, but what the heck – count your blessings. Think of maybe five things each day to be thankful for.

We need to celebrate the fact that we are still here. A little ragged round the edges, a little bruised. But still alive. No, more than alive, *living*.

Celebration is not just remembering the past, it is also affirming the present. We cannot truly celebrate if we are worrying about the future or fretting about the past. Try to be thankful for the now. In the last interview before his death, the British playwright Dennis Potter talked about the importance, the sacred nature, of the present moment:

> Things are both more trivial than they ever were and more important than they ever were, and the difference between the trivial and the important doesn't seem to matter. The nowness of everything is absolutely wondrous ... the glory of it, if you like, the comfort of it, the reassurance ... The fact that if you see the present tense, boy do you see it! And boy can you celebrate it![89]

A good thing can feel like a bad thing

I have Wi-Fi in the shed. *Wi-Fi*. I didn't expect that, it's a blessing from the Lord. I thought I was going to have to run some kind of cable, but reception is strong. It's a sign, I tell you, a sign.

Actually, it meant I could Skype my friend – let's call him Steve – and show him the shed. 'You've created a prayer chapel!' he said. I could sense the awe in his voice, even over Skype.

Steve is one of the guys who knows a lot about this dark night, spiritual formation business. Mainly because he's been through it himself. And he has spent a lot of time working with men's groups in spiritual formation – which is helping them to be more like Jesus.

'You get away with this idolatry all through the first stages of life,' he explained. 'Which is "I want God, but I want God on my terms." You're firmly in control. But the invitation of middle age, and of journeying throughout these crisis points, is learning you're not in control and that's OK. Actually God can be in control and you can trust God to be in control, because God genuinely has your best interests at heart.

'Spiritually, you have to make that journey of losing yourself to find yourself. And 99 per cent of us need a crisis, because you have to reach the end of your resources to discover grace and let that be the turning point. I mean, if you can do it without that, great. But it seems to be the natural order of things is some sort of crisis, a redundancy, an illness, a marriage break-up, an affair, whatever – something has to happen. That's why men buy cars and run off with secretaries and do all that stuff. It's the last vestiges of that ego-self saying, "Oh gosh, nothing's turning out as I thought it would." Which is a good thing, but it feels like a bad thing.'

We talked a bit about the 'disciplines' and which had helped him most.

'For me I guess there have been three disciplines that have been most important. In fact, I've observed these to lead to the most transformation in men. Silence and solitude is probably the number one. The real coming face to face with your demons. So, stop the background noise, stop listening to music all the time, stop watching TV. No, go to the silence. Those things that you're running away from – examine them. Look at them. Don't be scared by them. Name them for what they are.'

His second recommendation was interesting.

'I think second, fasting. Because pornography is such a huge draw and temptation. Without wanting to get all preachy or sound Victorian about it, there's something corrosive about that. And you hear sermons saying "Ooh it's dangerous, it objectifies women" – makes no difference. What makes a difference? Fasting does.'

'How does starving yourself help?' I asked. 'Does it make you too exhausted to turn on the computer or something?'

'The benefit of fasting is that if you do it, it just gives you a degree of confidence that says, you know what, I can control my desires, I don't have to act on them. That's really important in mid-life, where a lot of us men have areas of our lives that are out of control.'

His third recommendation was secrecy: doing things for others without needing recognition or approval or even being identified.

'Secrecy was one of those things which all of us in our men's group found important. I always say it appeals to my inner James Bond. It just does something very interesting to your own sense of confidence and well-being, and it sort of makes you feel good about yourself. It does exactly the opposite of what pornography does. Pornography gives you a quick fix, followed by this sort of general self-loathing. Secrecy does the absolute opposite. At the time of you doing these things it can be quite annoying or painful or inconvenient. But the long-term thing is that you start to feel quite good about yourself and your relationship with God.'

That is what these exercises are really all about. God does not call us into discipleship in order to humiliate us, or to make us even more aware of our own general crappiness. He calls us in out of friendship and love. And to be what we were intended to be. 'For we are what he has made us,' wrote Paul, 'created in Christ Jesus for good works, which God prepared beforehand to be our way of life' (Ephesians 2:10).

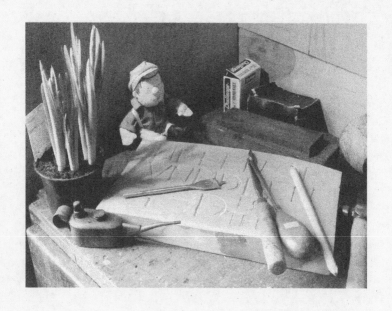

CONCLUSION

THE BRIGHT NIGHT OF THE SHED

Back to life

Outside the day is bright. Through the window which I put in at the end of the shed – another window from a skip – I can see a miniature, twisted, coiling willow tree. The Wife planted it many years ago in a pot in the garden and, as is her habit with plants, forgot to water it. By the end of summer, it was not so much a tree as an elaborate arrangement of very coiled, very dead sticks. I didn't chuck it, but planted it in the corner of a raised bed, because I thought its corkscrew branches, dead though they were, would at least provide some support for some peas I was trying to grow.

The peas didn't grow at all, but, amazingly, the willow came back to life. And this March morning it is covered with pale green lambs-tail catkins. Occasionally a robin comes and perches in the branches.

This morning, after prayers and before work, I dug compost into the bed where the willow tree is. I love compost. I love the idea of all that rubbish being transformed into new life. All the waste, all the scraps turn into magical, rich black soil. And all it takes is a bit of darkness and a bit of time.

Death and resurrection is the rule of the universe. Seeds fall into the ground, seeds *have* to fall into the ground.

Autumn must be undergone, winter endured, and spring anticipated. They're all about life.

On a shelf in the shed I put four objects: a small red oil-can, a children's soft toy, a postcard, and a vase of daffodils.

The red oil-can was owned by my grandfather. He was a watch repairer. A working-class farmer's son, he became an engineer, a motor mechanic. He could fix anything, could Pop. As a fireman in the war he caught TB in the Norwich blitz and nearly died. After that he took up watch repairing. I remember, as a small boy, being allowed to sit with him in his workshop – which was a shed out the back of his small terraced house. I can recall the smell of watch oil and the many tobacco tins full of useful bits and pieces. Maybe it's that youthful experience that lies behind this shed business. But the oil-can reminds me that the shed has to be a place of work and prayer. I will still do 'sheddy' stuff in here. One end of the shed will have a bench and tools and a place to make stuff, because without activity, without productivity, what's the point of discipleship?

The children's toy is a small doll of Percy the Park Keeper. It once belonged to one of my daughters when they were younger, but they never played with it much. In fact, I had to rescue him from them. I found him in among all the Barbies wearing nothing but his park keeper's hat and a pink cocktail dress. That was no way to treat a hero. I saved him from this life of transvestitism and gathered what I could find of the rest of his clothes (I never could find his left boot).

For those of you who don't know Percy the Park Keeper, as his name implies he looks after a park, assisted by a range of animals, including Fox, Badger, Rabbit, Squirrel, several Mice and possibly an Aardvark. Or not. I imagine, given the recent government cutbacks, he uses animals because they don't have to be paid the minimum wage.

Anyway, Percy has a shed. Probably the greatest shed in literature. Behind its welcoming green door and beneath its shingled roof there is everything a man could need: a desk, a rocking chair, pictures on the wall, drawers for everything important, a tin bath, a stove with a proper kettle, blue-and-white Cornishware mugs, and a bed.

A bed. Think about that. Percy *lives* in his shed. Now do you see why he's a hero?

In one episode, it is autumn and there are warnings of a storm. In his hut, Percy prepares for the rainy night. 'Just a drop of rain,' he tells himself. He tunes in his old valve radio to hear the weather forecast: 'Light breeze with a few showers,' says the lady announcer. Percy settles in bed with his mug of tea and a biscuit.

That night a massive storm hits the park. The next morning, Percy emerges from his shed to find a scene of devastation. The tree where the animals live has been blown over. 'Oh thump!' exclaims Percy. The rest of the episode shows how he helps the animals find a home and make it even better than before. But for me, the clear message of the episode was this: Percy survived the storm because he had a shed.

My life had been hit by a sudden storm. No one prepared me for it. When autumn arrived I was knocked flat. So maybe that was what this was all about. Building a refuge, a place to ride out the storm. We are all looking for something to get us through the storms of life. We all seek protection, a haven, a place where we can stay warm and safe.

Actually, maybe we're not so much like Percy as like the animals. The autumn storms lash us, they knock down the houses we thought were as solid as an oak tree. But for so many of us, these tempests are the only way to make us search for a new home. We cannot run away. Paradoxically, the only safe harbour is to be found by heading into the storm, and learning to trust in God.

Someone once said to the artist Edvard Munch – he of *The Scream* painting – 'You could rid yourself of your troubles.' Munch replied, 'They are part of me and my art. They are indistinguishable from me, and it would destroy my art. I want to keep those sufferings.'[90] I don't think we should necessarily keep hold of our sufferings. But we should honour them. Learn from them. Respect them. Listen to them. Every difficulty we go through, no matter how great or small, is a part of us and the great work of art that is our life.

Which brings me to the postcard. It's from the Tate Gallery. It's a picture of Epstein's sculpture *Jacob and the Angel*, of course.

After the river, after the wrestling, after the meeting with Esau, Jacob travels on and buys some land in Canaan. The Bible says that 'Jacob came safely to the city of Shechem.' The word translated 'safely' is *shelem*, which means 'complete, sound' or even 'uninjured'. The passage says that Jacob erected an altar there and called it 'El-Elohe-Israel', which means 'God, the God of Israel'. It's an acknowledgement of his changed allegiances. The God he met at the Jabbok was now his God. And his name was Israel.

Jacob came 'complete' and 'whole' to the city of Shechem. It was not the end of his troubles – far from it – but he was no longer the man he once had been. Or maybe he still was, a bit. Jacob ends his life with his sons in Egypt. 'Now the eyes of Israel were dim with age,' says the text, 'and he could not see well.' I've seen that somewhere before. And it gets even more déjà-vu-ish. Joseph brings his sons for a blessing from their grandfather. He tries to help his father by placing the boys in the proper position to receive the blessing, but 'Israel stretched out his right hand and laid it on the head of Ephraim, who was the younger, and his left hand on the head of Manasseh, crossing his hands, for Manasseh was the firstborn' (Genesis 48:13-14). Joseph tries to correct his father's 'mistake' and put the right hand on the eldest boy, but Jacob knows what he is doing. He knows the younger of the two boys will be greater. He's been involved with this sort of thing before.

The blessing he speaks over the boys is his story – or, at least, the story as he eventually came to understand it.

The God before whom my ancestors Abraham and Isaac walked,
the God who has been my shepherd all my life to this day,
the angel who has redeemed me from all harm, bless the boys;
and in them let my name be perpetuated, and the name of my ancestors Abraham and Isaac;
and let them grow into a multitude on the earth.

(Genesis 48:15-16)

'The angel who has redeemed me from all harm.' Who, I wonder, did Jacob have in mind here? Surely the figure in the stream. God defeated Jacob easily that night, and yet said that Jacob had 'prevailed'. Because what looked like a fight was actually a rescue; what looked like a defeat was really redemption.

The final object. A small bowl of daffodils. They are not flowering at the moment, they are still green, but spring is here and they will bloom soon.

Yes, spring is here. I began this journey in the russet days of autumn and end it in the green days of spring. Pretty soon now there will be swifts and swallows and house martins darting through the air. I was reading the other day about the restlessness of migratory birds. The scientist who discovered this called it *Zugunruhe* – 'movement anxiety'. It's innate in birds: both the need to migrate and the path which they should take is encoded into their very being. I believe that, at certain seasons of their life, human beings have *Zugunruhe*. The restless need to move to a different destination. That is what mid-life is all about.

And the destination? The theologian Karl Barth said, 'The goal of human life is not death, but resurrection.' That is the goal of the dark night as well. That is our call, our journey and our joy: we go willingly into the dark night because we know that it will lead to a new dawn.

And we are called to go out into the world with this good news. The shed started out as a refuge, a retreat, but it really is a place for recharging. The shed is a nice place to visit, but I wouldn't want to live there.

Easter is only a few days away now. In the Orthodox Church, the service on the night before Easter is called 'the bright night'. Gregory of Nyssa said, 'This night becomes brighter than the day.'[91] There are lines in the liturgy which contain this shining, incandescent promise of hope:

> O Christ, the Passover great and most holy!
> O Wisdom, Word and Power of God!
> Grant that we may more perfectly partake of Thee
> In the day of Thy Kingdom which knoweth no night.

Amen. Amen to that.

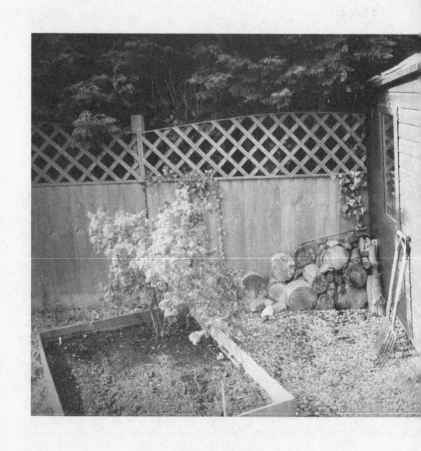

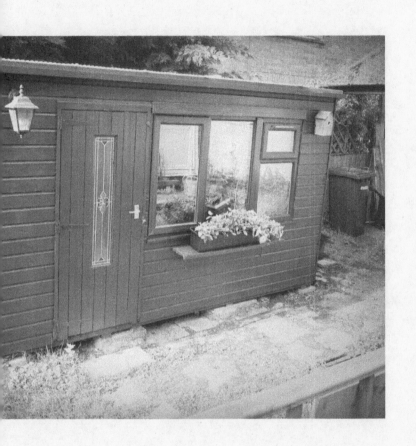

TOOLBOX

For more information on all this kind of stuff, plus links to interesting videos and many other goodies, visit www.darknightoftheshed.com.

There you can also pick up a Free Study Guide to accompany this book, containing discussion questions for small groups.

The books I've referenced in *The Dark Night of the Shed* are listed in the Notes. But here are the tools I've found most helpful.

On discipleship and the disciplines

Foster, R., *Celebration of Discipline: the Path to Spiritual Growth* (London: Hodder & Stoughton, 1980).

Hughes, G., *God of Surprises* (London: Darton, Longman & Todd, 1985).

Laird, M., *Into the Silent Land: The Practice of Contemplation* (London: Darton, Longman & Todd, 2006).

Nouwen, H., *The Return of the Prodigal Son* (London: Darton, Longman & Todd, 1994).

Wilkins, M., *Following the Master: Discipleship in the Steps of Jesus* (Grand Rapids: Zondervan, 1992).

Willard, D., *The Spirit of the Disciplines* (London: Hodder & Stoughton, 1996).

See also www.renovarelife.org, where you can find many resources, including some videos by Joe Davis which offer exercises to get you started.

General stuff about middle age

Bainbridge, D., *Middle Age: A Natural History* (London: Portobello Books, 2012).

Frankl, V., *Man's Search for Meaning* (London: Washington Square Press, 1985).

Layard, R., *Happiness: Lessons from a New Science* (London: Penguin, 2011).

Rohr, R., *Falling Upward: A Spirituality for the Two Halves of Life* (San Francisco; Chichester: Jossey-Bass, 2011).

Sheehy, G., *Understanding Men's Passages: Discovering the New Map of Men's Lives* (New York: Random House, 1998).

Some must-reads that don't fit in anywhere else

Bianco, M.W., and W. Nicholson, *The Velveteen Rabbit: Or How Toys Become Real* (London: Heinemann, 1922).

Booker, C., *The Seven Basic Plots: Why We Tell Stories* (London: Continuum, 2004).

Jansson, T., *Moominpappa at Sea* (London: Puffin Books, 1974).

John of the Cross and other luminaries of the dark night

John of the Cross, *Dark Night of the Soul* (London: Burns & Oates, 1976).

Ward, B., *The Desert Fathers: Sayings of the Early Christian Monks* (London: Penguin, 2003).

On Jacob's story

Sanford, J., *The Man who Wrestled with God: Light from the Old Testament on the Psychology of Individuation* (New York: Paulist Press, 1987).

For the Jung at heart

Bair, D., *Jung: A Biography* (London: Little, Brown, 2004).

Hollis, J., *Finding Meaning in the Second Half of Life* (New York: Gotham Books, 2006).

Johnson, R., *He: Understanding Masculine Psychology* (New York: Perennial Library, 1986).

Jung, C.G., *The Essential Jung* (London: Fontana, 1998).

Jung, C.G., *The Undiscovered Self* (New York: Signet, 2006).

Jung, C. G. and A. Jaffé, *Memories, Dreams, Reflections*, (London: Collins and Routledge & Kegan Paul, 1963)

Jung, C.G., W.S. Dell and C.F. Baynes, *Modern Man in Search of a Soul* (London: Ark Paperbacks, 1984).

Stevens, A., *Jung, A Very Short International* (Oxford: Oxford University Press, 2001)

On sheds

Hopkinson, F., *The Joy of Sheds* (London: Portico, 2012).

Thorburn, G., *Men and Sheds* (London: New Holland, 2002).

NOTES

1. Quoted in Max Olesker, 'How to Be a Man in 2015', *Observer*, 1 March 2015.
2. F. Hopkinson, *The Joy of Sheds* (London: Portico, 2012), p. 49.
3. H. Thoreau, *Walden; or, Life in the Woods* (Harmondsworth: Penguin, 1938), p. 80.
4. C. G. Jung and A Jaffé, *Memories, Dreams, Reflections* (London: Collins and Routledge & Kegan Paul, 1963), p. 184.
5. ibid., p. 214.
6. G. Sheehy, *Understanding Men's Passages: Discovering the New Map of Men's Lives* (New York: Random House, 1998), p. 9.
7. W. Langland, *Piers Plowman*, XII, 7 (Harmondsworth: Penguin, 1966), p. 141.
8. J. Sanford, *The Man who Wrestled with God: Light from the Old Testament on the Psychology of Individuation* (New York: Paulist Press, 1987), p. 21.
9. T. Jansson, *Moominpappa at Sea* (London: Puffin Books, 1974), p. 7.
10. ibid., p. 25.
11. See John of the Cross, *Dark Night of the Soul* (London: Burns & Oates, 1976), p. 98.
12. ibid., p. 64.

13. Translated by R.O. Faulkner in W.K. Simpson (ed.), *The Literature of Ancient Egypt* (New Haven; London: Yale University Press, 1973), pp. 201-9.

14. C. Booker, *The Seven Basic Plots: Why We Tell Stories* (London: *Continuum*, 2004)

15. Sheehy, *Understanding Men's Passages*, p. 45.

16. L. Segal, *Out of Time* (London: Verso Books, 2013), p. 5.

17. On all the theories, see D. Bainbridge, *Middle Age: A Natural History* (London: Portobello Books, 2012), p. 27.

18. Quoted in Segal, *Out of Time*, p. 176.

19. Sheehy, *Understanding Men's Passages*, p. 97.

20. R. Layard, *Happiness: Lessons from a New Science* (London: Penguin, 2011), p. 29.

21. ibid., p. 33.

22. ibid., p. 35.

23. Statistics from the International Stress Management Association, http://www.isma.org.uk/

24. Quoted in J. Hollis, *Finding Meaning in the Second Half of Life* (New York: Gotham Books, 2006), p. 170.

25. ibid., pp. 149-50.

26. 'Finally, Some Actual Stats on Internet Porn', Gizmodo, http://gizmodo.com/5552899/finally-some-actual-stats-on-internet-porn.

27. Hopkinson, *The Joy of Sheds*, p. 23.

28. Quoted in Segal, *Out of Time*, p. 75.

29. C.G. Jung, W.S. Dell and C.F. Baynes, *Modern Man in Search of a Soul* (London: Ark Paperbacks, 1984), p. 127.

30. Jung described his father: 'As a country parson he had lapsed into a sort of sentimental idealism and into reminiscences of his golden student days, continued to smoke a long student's pipe, and discovered that his marriage was not all he had imagined it to be. He did a great deal of good – far too

much – and as a result was usually irritable.' On all this, see Jung and Jaffé, *Memories, Dreams, Reflections*, pp. 95ff.

31. Quoted on http://www.damaris.org/film-and-bible-blog/1285.

32. Quoted in Hollis, *Finding Meaning in the Second Half of Life*, p. 219.

33. G. Hughes, *God of Surprises* (London: Darton, Longman & Todd, 1985), p. 71.

34. Jung, *Modern Man in Search of a Soul*, p. 125.

35. R. Rohr, *Falling Upward: A Spirituality for the Two Halves of Life* (San Francisco; Chichester: Jossey-Bass, 2011), p. 32.

36. From *Symbols of Transformation*, quoted in C. Booker, *The Seven Basic Plots*, p. 237.

37. V. Hamilton, *The Book of Genesis* (Grand Rapids: William B. Eerdmans, 1990), p. 329.

38. Sanford, *The Man who Wrestled with God*, p. 40.

39. F. Spufford, *Unapologetic* (London: Faber & Faber, 2013), p. 222.

40. H. Nouwen, *The Return of the Prodigal Son* (London: Darton, Longman & Todd, 1994), p. 107.

41. Spufford, *Unapologetic*, p. 8.

42. G. Orwell, *The Collected Essays, Journalism and Letters of George Orwell* (Harmondsworth: Penguin, 1970), vol. 4, p. 579.

43. Quoted in R. Rohr, *Simplicity: The Freedom of Letting Go* (New York: Crossroad Roundhouse, 2003), p. 173.

44. Rohr, *Falling Upward*, p. 72.

45. W. Brueggemann, *Genesis* (Atlanta: John Knox Press, 1982), p. 268.

46. A. Bloom, *School for Prayer* (London, Libra Books, 1970), p. 11.

47. Abba Poemen in B. Ward, *The Desert Fathers: Sayings of the Early Christian Monks* (London: Penguin, 2003), p. 158.

48. D. Willard, *The Divine Conspiracy: Rediscovering Our Hidden Life in God* (London: Fount, 1998), p. 224.

49. Sanford, *The Man who Wrestled with God*, p. 25.

50. Hollis, *Finding Meaning in the Second Half of Life*, p. 216.

51. See 'Repentance' in *New International Dictionary of New Testament Theology* (Grand Rapids: Zondervan, 2014), pp. 357-8.

52. See G. Thorburn, *Men and Sheds* (London: New Holland, 2002).

53. Hughes, *God of Surprises*, p. 116.

54. Nouwen, *The Return of the Prodigal Son*.

55. *The Peloponnesian War*, book 1, 118, in Thucydides, *History of the Peloponnesian War* (Harmondsworth: Penguin Books, 1972), p. 103.

56. Augustine, *Confessions* (Oxford: Oxford University Press, 1998), p. 201.

57. Quoted in M. Laird, *Into the Silent Land: The Practice of Contemplation* (London: Darton, Longman & Todd, 2006), p. 9.

58. Laird, *Into the Silent Land*, p. 15.

59. John of the Cross, *Living Flame*, stanza 3, para 6.

60. Sanford, *The Man who Wrestled with God*, p. 21.

61. C.G. Jung and R.F.C. Hull, *The Development of Personality*, *Collected Works*, vol. 17 (London: Routledge & Kegan Paul, 2014), para 289, p. 300.

62. Ward, *The Desert Fathers*, pp. 3-4.

63. M.W. Bianco and W. Nicholson, *The Velveteen Rabbit: Or How Toys Become Real* (London: Heinemann, 1922), pp. 3-4.

64. D. Willard, *The Divine Conspiracy: Rediscovering our Hidden Life in God* (London: Fount, 1998), p. 224.

65. The saying is found in Codex D version of Luke and is one of

the *agrapha*, or sayings of Jesus recorded outside the canonical text of the New Testament. The scholar Jeremias says of this saying that 'The case for its authenticity is as strong as the improbability of its spuriousness.' Which now I've typed it, I'm not sure what he means. But he argues for a Palestinian provenance and sees it as a typically Jesus-like antithesis. See J. Jeremias, *Unknown Sayings of Jesus* (London: SPCK, 1957), pp. 49-54. Similarly, in his comprehensive collection *The Hidden Sayings of Jesus*, William Morrice gives this story an A rating. See W.G. Morrice, *Hidden Sayings of Jesus: Words Attributed to Jesus Outside the Four Gospels* (London: SPCK, 1997), p. 34. That there are more sayings around should not surprise us. Luke says that many others set out to make a record of Jesus' life and John admitted he had to be selective in his choice of material (John 21:25).

66. M. Wilkins, *Following the Master: Discipleship in the Steps of Jesus* (Grand Rapids: Zondervan, 1992), p. 60.

67. The Ignatius references are *Eph.* 1.1.3, 10.3.2, *Trall.* 1.2.3 and *Phld.* 7.2.4. For Polycarp see *The Martyrdom of Polycarp*, 17.3.2.

68. D. Willard, *The Divine Conspiracy*, p. 29.

69. Ward, *The Desert Fathers*, p. 5.

70. R. Foster, *Celebration of Discipline: The Path to Spiritual Growth* (London: Hodder & Stoughton, 1980), p. 85.

71. Ward, *The Desert Fathers*, p. 10.

72. H. Nouwen, *The Way of the Heart: Desert Spirituality and Contemporary Ministry* (London: Darton, Longman & Todd, 1981), p. 31.

73. See F. Gros, *A Philosophy of Walking* (London: Verso, 2014), p. 3.

74. J. Burnside, 'Alone', *London Review of Books*, 9 February 2012, p. 24.

75. Sanford, *The Man who Wrestled with God*, p. 39.

76. Karl Banth, 'The Strange New World Within the Bible' in, *The Word of God and the Word of Man*, trans. Douglas Horton (New York: Harper & Row, 1957), p. 28

77. See Burrow, quoted in S. Tugwell, *Ways of Imperfection: An Exploration of Christian Spirituality* (London: Darton, Longman & Todd, 1984), p. 106.

78. Alice Walker, 'Why I'm Joining the Freedom Flotilla to Gaza', *Guardian*, 25 June 2011.

79. http://www.bbc.co.uk/news/magazine-30849473.

80. Ward, *The Desert Fathers*, p. 10.

81. Foster, *Celebration of Discipline*, p. 69.

82. M.W. Holmes, *The Apostolic Fathers: Greek Texts and English Translations* (Grand Rapids: Baker Academic, 2007), pp. 289, 575.

83. D. Willard, *The Spirit of the Disciplines* (London: Hodder & Stoughton, 1996), p. 172.

84. See *Letter of His Holiness Pope John Paul II to Artists*, 1999, at http://w2.vatican.va/content/john-paul-ii/en/letters /1999/documents/hf_jp-ii_let_23041999_artists.html.

85. Hughes, *God of Surprises*, p. 3.

86. A. Schmemann, *The World as Sacrament* (London: Darton, Longman & Todd, 1966), p. 26.

87. See M. Ricard, *The Art of Meditation* (London: Atlantic, 2010), p. 23.

88. M. Gaffney, *Flourishing* (London: Penguin, 2012), p. 77.

89. ibid., p. 362.

90. Layard, *Happiness*, p. 220.

91. Schmemann, *The World as Sacrament*, pp. 70-71.

THANKS

All books are the products of many influences and inputs, but this book in particular could not have come about without the help of many people. Especial thanks are due to all of the following people.

All my many friends and teachers on the Renovaré Institute Spiritual Formation course, especially Gary Moon and Trevor Hudson.

My friends and fellow wise old men Martin Cavender and my brother David. And thanks to all the Steves I have spoken to, especially the two doctors.

Joe Davis for his constant encouragement and support. Check out his videos at www.renovarelife.org.

All those in my church community at St Leonards, Eynsham. Mainly for putting up with me. See you in the shed!

Ian Metcalfe and the team at Hodder for endless patience and support.

My children, Lily, Madeleine and Martha, for keeping me grounded and occasionally even looking interested.

And most of all, to The Wife. You know I couldn't do any of this without you, don't you?

www.darknightoftheshed.com

Visit www.darknightoftheshed.com for more resources, ideas, inspiration, and all manner of digital shediness.

And you can download a FREE Study Guide to accompany this book, containing discussion questions for small groups.

It's specially designed for you and some friends to discuss over a cup of tea in your shed, or a pint down the pub.

(Please note: friends, tea and beer are not provided.)

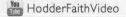